Practical Meat Science

Practical Meat Science

Ashim Kumar Biswas
Senior Scientist (LPT)
Division of Post-Harvest Technology, ICAR-CARI,
Izatnagar, Bareilly-243122 (U.P.)
E-mail: biswaslpt@gmail.com

Prabhat Kumar Mandal
Associate Professor
Department of Livestock Products Technology,
Rajiv Gandhi Institute of Veterinary
Education and Research, Kurumbapet,
Puducherry-605009
E-mail: mandalpkm@gmail.com

SSPH

SATISH SERIAL PUBLISHING HOUSE
403, Express Tower, Commercial Complex
Azadpur, Delhi-110033 (India)
Phone : 011-27672852, Fax : 91-11-27672046
e-mail : info@satishserial.com, hkjain1975@yahoo.com
Website : www.satishserial.com

Published by :

SATISH SERIAL PUBLISHING HOUSE

403, Express Tower, Commercial Complex, Azadpur, Delhi-110033 (INDIA)
Phone : 011-27672852 Fax : 91-11-27672046
E-mail : info@satishserial.com, hkjain1975@yahoo.com

ISBN 978-93-86200-39-6

Composed, Designed & Printed in India

About the Authors

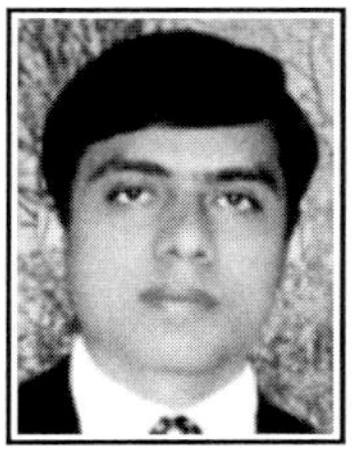

Dr. Ashim Kumar Biswas Born on 05th March 1978 in West Bengal, got BVSc & AH from WBUA& FSc, Kolkata in 2000, MVSc (in 2002) and PhD (in 2005) in Livestock Products Technology from, Indian Veterinary Research Institute, Izatnagar. In 2005, he joined as Assistant Professor in the Department of LPT, SKUAST-Jammu. On Feb 2007, he joined as Assistant Professor in the Department of LPT, GADVASU, Ludhiana. Presently he is serving as Senior Scientist in Division of Post-Harvest Technology at Central Avian Research Institute (ICAR), Izatnagar. He has more than 150 publications in his credit.

His main achievements in research is relating to evaluation of export buffalo meat for quality, development of enrobed meat products, restructured buffalo meat blocks, functional based & shelf stable value added meat products. His research also focused on development and validation of HPLC methodologies for detection of pesticide and veterinary drug residues in meat and meat products. He also standardized molecular techniques (PCR) for the detection of bacterial pathogens in livestock products. He teaches several LPT courses at the University and guides many undergraduate and postgraduate students since 2006. He handled or currently handling several research projects and grants funded by MFPI, DST, RKVY (Govt. of India), ICAR, etc in the capacity of PI and Co-PI.

He has Co-edited an advance reference book "Animal Products Technology" and author of a text book "Poultry, Egg and Fish Processing Technology" for PG level and another text book "Abattoir, Byproducts and Wool" for U. G Veterinary students. Dr. Biswas is a fellow of Indian Poultry Science Association, NAAS Associate, Associate Editor, Journal of Meat Science and Indian Journal of Poultry Science.

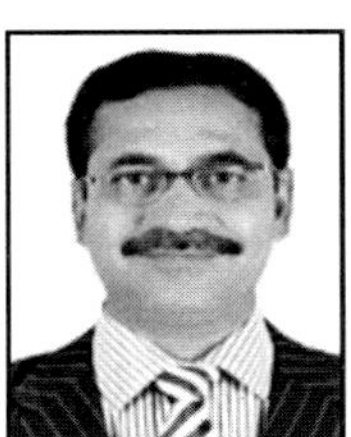

Dr. Prabhat Kumar Mandal was born in 1967 in West Bengal, got BVSc & AH from Bidhan Chandra Krishi Viswavidyalaya, Kolkata, in 1991 and did his MVSc & PhD majoring in Livestock Products Technology from Indian Veterinary Research Institute, Izatnagar in the year 1993 and 1996, respectively. He is a recipient of National Scholarship from GOI (1984-1991), JRF (1991–1993) and SRF (1993–1996) from IVRI. He worked for a short period (1996) as Scientist (ARS) in ICAR and then joined as Assistant Professor in Dept of LPT in September 1996, in Rajiv Gandhi College of Veterinary and Animal Sciences, Pondicherry. He was promoted as Associate Professor in March, 2005 and Associate Professor, Senior Grade from March, 2008.

Dr. Mandal is teaching several UG and PG courses related to meat science and engaged in research on Meat Science and Technology/Livestock Products Technology since last 20 years. His research achievements include development of chicken meat balls from spent hen meat, utilization of blood protein isolates in sausages and cakes, development of poultry products utilizing edible byproducts, low fat restructured chicken block and using gizzard and natural preservatives. Presently he is working on development of functional meat foods with natural preservatives. Dr. Mandal has more than 150 publications in his credit.

He worked as Visiting Professor in Hankyong National Univrsity, South Korea and Konkuk University, Seoul from March, 2008 to February, 2010. He was Associate Editor/Editor, Journal of Meat Science published by IMSA since 2003-13. Presently Dr. Mandal is Editor-in-Chief of International Journal of Meat Science and Journal of Meat Science. He has Edited an advance reference book "Animal Products Technology" and co-author of a text book "Poultry, Egg and Fish Processing Technology" for PG level and another text book "Abattoir, Byproducts and Wool" for U. G. Veterinary students. Dr. Mandal is a Fellow of Indian Poultry Science Association and Indian Meat Science Association.

Preface

Foods of animal origin with high biological value are very important source of animal proteins and other most important nutrients for life sustenance of human being. There is heavy demand for the muscle foods and the consumers are very much aware about the quality aspects and their consequences on health. Accordingly lots of researches are going on in this area to provide quality meat and meat products. There is urgent need for stringent quality control of such foods especially with the implementation of Food Safety and Standard Act, 2006. Large numbers of trained scientific work force are required to conduct regular inspection and analysis of the muscle foods by the Food Safety and Standard Authority of India for this purpose. To conduct proper inspection and quality analysis of muscle foods and for the teaching and research community there is need for a practical book for ready reference. We both have long teaching and research experience which has helped us to compile this book based on experience.

The book has ten different sections covering every aspects of quality evaluation for muscle foods. Section-I is about general instructions, Section-II covering analysis of chemical composition of muscle foods for protein, fats, fibre and minerals. Section-III deals with evaluation of functional quality of meat including water holding capacity, muscle fibre diameter, sarcomere length, myofibrillar fragmentation index, emulsion stability, emulsifying capacity, instrumental textural value, muscle fiber typing. Section IV is about assessment of keeping quality of meat for pH, extract release volume, water activity, lipid quality, protein quality, acidity, glycogen content, microbial quality and sensory evaluation.

Section-V for measuring meat colour using of lovibond tintometer and spectrophotometer. Section-VI for determination of functional compounds in meat viz. antioxidative activity, different bioactive compounds, different vitamins; Section-VII about molecular techniques for detection of tenderizing enzymes in meat. Section-VIII on monitoring of food additives and chemical residues using HPLC; Section -IX for rapid identification of certain meat quality parameters. Section-X covers methods for species differentiation for meat including chemical, serological and molecular techniques

The book is prepared for handy reference with easy to understand language and précised steps for the procedure to conduct analysis of every quality parameters. The principle behind every method and the requirements to conduct the tests are explained in very simple points. The methods are compiled from the standard resources viz, books, journal, manuals, thesis etc and duly cited in respective sections. We hope this Book will be very much useful to the Post graduate students, Teachers, Researchers/Scientists and Food Inspectors related to the muscle foods.

Ashim Kumar Biswas
Prabhat Kumar Mandal

Contents

About the Authors .... *v*
Preface .... *vii*

I. **General Instructions** **1**
1. Introduction 1
2. Laboratory safety 2
3. Cleaning laboratory wares 2
4. Preparation of cleaning solution 3
5. Laboratory instruction 3
6. Orientation and use of a compound microscope 4
7. Use of common bacteriological apparatus 6
8. Cleaning and sterilization 6
9. Methods of preparing chemical solutions 7
10. Sampling procedure 8

II. **Analysis of Chemical Composition of Muscle Foods** **11**
1. Moisture 11
1.1 Preparation of sample 12
1.2 Methods 12
2. Protein 16
2.1 Crude protein 16
2.2 Sarcoplasmic proteins 23
2.3 Myofibrillar proteins 24
2.4 Stromal proteins (Acid soluble protein) 24
2.5 Collagen (Hydroxyproline estimation) 25
3. Lipid analysis 27
3.1 Ether extracts (Soxhlet method) 28

3.2 Total lipids (Gravimetric method) 29
3.3 Total phospholipids 29
3.4 Total cholesterol 31
3.5 Fatty acid profile (GLC method) 33
3.6 Iodine value 34
3.7 Saponification number 35
4. Crude fibre 36
4.1 Principle 36
4.2 Apparatus and chemicals 36
4.3 Procedure 36
5. Mineral determination 37
5.1 Methods of ashing 38

III. **Evaluation of Functional Quality of Meat 43**
1. Water holding capacity (WHC) 43
1.1 Centrifugal method 43
1.2 Filter paper press method 44
2. Muscle fibre diameter (Microscopic method) 44
2.1 Method I 45
Method II (Formalin fixing method) 45
3. Measurement of sarcomere length (Microscopic method) 46
3.1 Principle 46
3.2 Apparatus and chemicals 46
3.3 Procedure 47
4. Myofibrillar fragmentation index (MFI) 47
4.1 Method I (Phosphate-EDTA method) 47
Method II (Sucrose-KCl method) 48
5. Emulsion stability (ES) 49
5.1 Principle 49
5.2 Apparatus and chemicals/solvents 49
5.3 Procedure 49

6. Emulsifying capacity 50
6.1 Principle 50
6.2 Apparatus and chemicals/solvents 50
6.3 Procedure 50
7. Determination of instrumentation textural value 51
7.1 Warner-Bratzler/Kramer shear force value 51
7.2 Texture profile analysis (TPA) 52
8. Muscle fiber typing (Combined staining for identifying muscle fiber types) 54
8.1 Principle 54
8.2 Solutions 54
8.3 Staining sequence 55
8.4 Results 55
References 56

IV. **Assessment of Keeping Quality of Meat 57**
1. pH 57
1.1 Principle 58
1.2 Apparatus and chemicals 58
1.3 Procedure 58
2. Extract release volume (ERV) 59
2.1 Principle 59
2.2 Apparatus and chemicals 59
2.3 Procedure 59
3. Water activity (a_w) 60
3.1 Principle 60
3.2 Apparatus, raw materials and chemicals 60
3.3 Procedure 60
4. Lipid quality 60
4.1 Thiobrbituric acid reacting substance (TBARS) value 61
4.2 Free fatty acids (FFAs) 64

4.3 Peroxide value (PV) 64
4.4 Acid value 65
5. Protein quality 66
5.1 Protein oxidation 66
5.2 Tyrosine value 67
5.3 Free amino acid content 68
5.4 Total volatile nitrogen (TVN) 69
6. Estimation of acidity 70
6.1 Total acidity (Lactic acid) 70
6.2 Titrable acidity (TA) 71
7. Glycogen content 72
7.1 Principle 73
7.2 Apparatus and chemicals 73
7.3 Procedure 73
8. Microbial quality 75
8.1 Properties of good sample 75
8.2 Microbial sampling of meat/poultry products 76
8.3 Preparation of homogenate and serial dilution 77
9. Sensory evaluation 80
9.1 Difference between sensory and organoleptic evaluation 80
9.2 Requirements of testing conditions for sensory evaluation 81
9.3 Sensory panel room 82
9.4 Time of taste: Depends upon the sample 83
9.5 Development of panel 83
9.6 Preparation and presentation of samples 87
9.7 Sensory evaluation methods 87
9.8 Difference test/Descriptive test 89
References 89

V. **Methods for Exploration of Meat Colour** **91**

1. Use of Lovibond tintometer 92

1.1 Principle 92

1.2 Apparatus and materials 92

1.3 Procedure 93

2. Spectrophotometric method 94

2.1. Estimation of total meat pigments (Myoglobin) 94

2.2. Metmyoglobin content 95

2.3. Nitroso pigment (Cured meat products) 96

References 97

VI. **Methods for Determination of Functional Compounds in Meat Products** **99**

1. Antioxidant activity 99

1.1 DPPH (1,1-diphenyl-2-picrylhydrazyl) radical scavenging activity 100

1.2 ABTS (2-2-azinobis-3 ethylbenthiazoline-6-sulphonic acid) radical cation activity 101

1.3 Superoxide anion scavenging activity (SASA) 103

2. Bioactive compound 105

2.1 Total phenolics 105

2.2 Total flavonoids 106

2.3 Gallic acid 107

2.4 Reutin 108

3. Vitamins 108

3.1 β-carotene 108

3.2 α-tocopherol acetate (Vitamin E) 109

3.3 Ascorbic acid (Vitamin C) 110

References 111

VII. **Techniques for Detection of Tenderizing Enzymes in Meat** **113**

1. μ- and m-calpains (Casein zymography method) 113
   1.1 Principle 113
   1.2 Apparatus and reagents 114
   1.3 Procedure 115
2. Calpains and calpastatin 116
   2.1 SDS-PAGE method 116
   2.2 Biochemical test 120
3. Cathepsin B, D and H 123
   3.1 Apparatus and chemicals 123
   3.2 Procedure 123
4. ATPase activity 124
   4.1 Principle 124
   4.2 Equipment 124
   4.3 Reagents 124
   References 125

VIII. **Methods for Monitoring of Food Additives and Chemical Residues** **127**

1. Chemical method for identification of important food additives 127
   1.1 Nitrate (Xylenol method) 127
   1.2 Nitrites 130
   1.3 Salt and chlorides 132
   1.4 Nitrosamines 135
   1.5 Phosphates and residual phosphates 138
2. HPLC method for identification of veterinary drug residues 141
   2.1 Trimethoprim and sulfonamides 141
   2.2 Apparatus, raw materials and chemicals 142
   2.3 Procedure 143

2.4 Tetracycline, oxytetracycline and chlortetracyline 145
3. HPLC method for identification of pesticide residues 150
3.1 Carbaryl 150
3.2 Cyphermethrin and deltamethrin 154
References 159

IX. **Rapid Test for Identification of Meat Quality 161**
1. Physical examination of meat 161
2. Test for inefficiency of bleeding (Malachite green test) 161
2.1 Principle 161
2.2 Requirements 162
2.3 Procedure 162
3. Resazurin test (Dye reduction test) 162
3.1 Background 162
3.2 Requirements 162
3.3 Procedure 163
4. Rimington and fowrie test (Jaundice test) 164
5. Nitrazine-yellow test 164
6. Water protein ratio 164
7. Test for abnormal odour 165
7.1 Boiling test 165
7.2 Frying test 165
8. Copper sulphate test 165
9. Meat swelling capacity 165
10. Differentiation of chilled and thawed frozen meat 166
10.1 Background 166
10.2 Preparation of meat press juice 166

X. **Methods for Species Differentiation of Meat 169**
1. Physical techniques 170

2. Anatomical techniques 172
2.1 Dentition 172
2.2 Bone percentage of carcass 173
2.3 Ribs on thorax 173
2.4 Characteristics of long bones 173
3. Histological techniques 174
4. Chemical techniques 174
5. Molecular techniques (PCR based techniques) 175
5.1 Restriction fragment length polymorphism (RFLP) 175
5.2 Species-specific PCR 178
5.3 Multiplex PCR 180
5.4 Forensically information nucleotide sequencing (FINS) 182
Referemces 184

Chapter I

General Instructions

1. Introduction

Analysis of muscle food requires due care since it is an interdisciplinary science that integrates systematically the biochemistry, muscle biology, physics and mathematical sciences. So efforts are require good laboratory habits while working in the labs. Some instructions for working in the laboratory are given here and it is advised to read them carefully before they begin their work in the laboratory.

- Maintain the laboratory floor, benches, tabletops and other surfaces clean.
- Tools, equipment, and materials shall be stored in a orderly manner.
- Apparatus to be used should be neat and clean.
- Rubber bulb should be used while using glass pipette.
- The small amount of liquid remaining in the pipette should not be blown out in standardizing the pipettes; allowance is always made for this. However, a frosted ring near the top of recently manufactured pipettes indicates that the last drop is to be blown out.
- As a general rule, the heating of calibrated equipment should be avoided. Rapid cooling can change the glass structure and cause changes in volume.
- The top of cabinets and lockers should be kept free of cartons, bottles and miscellaneous items.
- Each work area and storage space should be examined for safety and convenience.

- Unlabelled or poorly labelled reagents or materials should be discarded.

2. Laboratory safety

- Laboratory should be well ventilated and fitted with exhaust fans for effective removal of fumes.
- Use apron and other devices like gloves, goggles etc depending upon the material to be handled.
- Do not add water to acids. Keep acids off skin ad protect eyes from spattering. If acids are spilled on the skin, wash off immediately with tap water. Gaseous nitrogen oxides from HNO_3 can cause severe lung damage. Copious flow of fumes is there when both concentrated HNO_3 and HCI are mixed together.
- If acid falls on clothes, neutralize the same with few drops of dilute ammonia solution or some other weak alkali solution.
- If acid spills on the floor or the table, neutralize it with some weak alkali and wipe off with duster.
- If you happen to suck acid into your mouth during pipetting, wash your mouth quickly with water and then rinse with a weak solution of washing soda.
- Use fume hood to protect against any type of fumes.
- Avoid use of equipments for purposes other than intended.
- Strong acids and other corrosive chemicals should be stored in cabinets lined with lead and located near a fume hood and emergency shower.
- Volatile corrosive chemicals should be protected from heat.
- Flammable liquids stored in the laboratory may be limited to no more than one day's supply.

3. Cleaning laboratory wares

- The glass and porcelain wares should be thoroughly washed with some detergent then these should be extensively rinsed with tap water followed by further rinsing with distilled water.
- If a grease film remains after cleaning with detergent, a cleaning solution consisting of sodium or potassium dichromate in

concentrated sulphuric acid may be used. After this rinsing is necessary in order to remove the last traces of dichromate ions, which adhere strongly to glass or porcelain surface.

4. Preparation of cleaning solution

- Chromic acid solution (80g potassium dichromate in 300 mL water + 460 mL of concentrated sulphuric acid) for 6-8 h before detergent cleaning.

5. Laboratory instructions

- Remember that you are in a microbiological laboratory and are working with microbes, some of which may be capable of producing disease. Therefore, take extreme care in handling the cultures, slides and other materials, which you may use or come in contact in the laboratory.
- Handover all used slides and cover glasses to the attendant or discard them in the specific container.
- Avoid spillage of materials or stains.
- Wash your hands before you leave the laboratory.
- In case of an accident, please bring it to the attention of the instructor.
- Take extreme care while you handle the Microscope you will be held responsible for any damage to the Microscope.
- If you have used an oil immersion lens make sure that you have cleaned the lens with Xylene before you return the instrument.
- Always make it a rule to flame the inoculating needle before and after use. Also, always open a culture tube or flask near the flame.
- The instruction book is provided so that you can prepare and plan your laboratory work. Therefore, read the instructions carefully before you come to the laboratory. Your laboratory report on the exercise you perform should be submitted for evaluation before performing the succeeding exercise.
- Use a white laboratory coat/apron and a separate piece of cloth to clean up the workbench.

6. Orientation and use of a compound microscope

- A compound microscope is defined as a magnifying optical instrument consisting of two lens systems, the objective and the ocular.
- Parts of a Microscope: Base, arm, inclination joint, mechanical clips, condenser with diaphragm, mirror or light source, body tube, revolving nose piece, objectives, draw tube, coarse and fine adjustments and eye piece.
- Magnifying power of a Microscope: Magnifying power of the objective X Magnifying power of the eye piece.

6.1 Use of low power objective

6.1.1 Preparation of a wet mount

- Take a clean slide (Clean the slide by washing with detergent powder and wiping with a clean piece of cloth.
- Make it grease free by passing over the flame for two to three times.
- Place a drop of the suspension on the glass slide.
- Place the cover slip over the drop taking care to avoid any air bubbles.
- Set the microscope on the table with the mirror facing the lamp or outside light.

6.1.2 Preliminary focusing and use of low power objective

- Arrange the microscope and the mirror so that the light coming up from the mirror passes through the slide.
- Place the wet mount on the stage of the microscope.
- Swing the low power objective into position. Make certain that it does not touch the cover slip.
- Turn the coarse adjustment until the object appears in approximate focus. The distance between the bottom lens of the objective and the object when in focus is called the working distance. Higher the magnification, smaller the working distance.

- Use the fine adjustment to sharpen the focus. Once the object is seen, do not use the coarse adjustment.
- Draw a picture of the specimen as it appears under the low power objective and mention the magnification.
- Use of condenser and mirror: Proper lighting is of primary importance to successful microscopy and this can be obtained by appropriate adjustment of the condenser and the mirror. Move the condenser all the way down slowly. Describe the effect of moving the condenser.
- While looking through the eye piece move the metal handle which adjusts the diaphragm and get familiar with the functions of Iris diaphragm.

6.2 Use of medium power objective

Protozoa : These are unicellular microorganisms which are non-photosynthetic, and mostly motile.

Algae : These are unicellular or multicellular, photosynthetic, and motile or non-motile microorganisms.

Yeast : They are unicellular fungi, divide mostly by budding.

6.2.1 Procedure

- Prepare a wet mount of the given samples on a clean slide.
- First examine under low power objective and describe the object.
- Swing the medium power in position taking care that it does not touch the cover slip and then sharpen the focus with fix adjustment knob only.
- Make the labelled diagram. Mention the magnification of the object.

6.3 Use of oil immersion objective

- In low and medium power objectives, the light passes from denser medium (glass) to a rarer medium (air) and so refracts away from its path. By placing a drop of oil whose refractive index is equal to that of glass, more light is made to pass through the object to the objective with the result the object will be seen brighter. The resolution will also be more.

- Resolving power of the microscope is the ability of the objective to differentiate between two objects, which are placed very near to each other, and it depends on the wavelength of the light used for observing the object.

7. Use of common bacteriological apparatus

- Hot Air Oven: Double jacketed, dry air circulated with thermostatic control, glasswares are sterilized using hot air oven at 160°C for 2.5h or at 180°C for 1.5 h. Temperature of 160°C is preferred to 180°C to prevent charring.
- Autoclave: Used for sterilization of media, rubber and plastic wares by use of moist heat at 15 lbs pressure or 121°C for 15 min; better heat penetration kills spore formers.
- Incubator: Range of temperature is 25 to 100°C. Used for incubating the Petri plates inoculated with test samples, operated at 35°C for 24-48 h for APC or SPC. It is thermostatically controlled.
- BOD Incubator: It is with temperature, and humidity control, can be used in wider range of temperature, from refrigerating or chilling temperature to higher temperature up to 100°C

8. Cleaning and sterilization

- Cleaning and sterilization of glasswares are of utmost importance to obtain accurate microbial analysis.
- Cleaning is done by using warm (50-55°C) detergent solution (1% washing soda or trisodium phosphate) using a brush.
- For cleaning the sticky materials from pipettes, these are immersed in chromic acid solution (80g potassium dichromate in 300 mL water + 460 mL of concentrated sulphuric acid) for 6 - 8 h before detergent cleaning.
- Petri plates and pipettes are kept in respective containers before putting in a hot air oven.
- Flasks and bottles can be directly kept inside the oven.
- In case of glass stopper bottles, a piece of paper should be inserted in the mouth of the bottle prior to sterilization to prevent jamming.

- After putting the oven on, wait for it to achieve a temperature of 160-180°C. Maintain this temperature for 2-2.5 h. After this, gradually cool down for about 2h.
- Do not open the oven immediately after switching off, as it causes serious breakage.

Notes:

- Cleaning solution should be discharged when it acquired green colour of chromium ion.
- Cleaning solution is most effective when warmed up to about 70°C. At this temperature it rapidly attacks plant and animal matter and thus it is potentially a dangerous preparation.
- Spillage, if occurs, should be cleaned with water.

9. Methods of preparing chemical solutions

9.1 Percent solution

- Percent solution contains 1 gram of the substance in 100 ml of the solvent. If v/v is given, it means 1 ml in 100 ml of solvent.

  W / V % is the number of grams of the substance in 100 ml of the solution.

  V / V % is the number of ml of the substance in 100 ml of the solution.

9.2 Normal solution (N)

- It is defined as the number of gram equivalents of a substance in one liter of a solution e.g. the equivalent weight of NaOH is 40, so 40 g in 1 liter of solution is 1N NaOH solution.

9.3 Molarity

- It is defined as the number of moles of the substance in one liter of the solution (1 mole means one gram molecular weight in the case of a molecular, one gram atomic weight in the case of an atom, one gram ionic weight in the case of an ion).

E.g. 1 M NaOH contains 40 g sodium hydroxide in one litre of solution, 1 mM NaOH contains 40 milligrams sodium hydroxide in one liter solution.

9.4 Molality

- It is defined as number of moles of the substance in 1000 g of solvent.

10. Sampling procedure

- In the analysis of meat and meat products, the most important step is the preparation of a representative sample.
- A sample is a small portion taken from a bulk of material for examination.
- The purpose of sampling is to obtain representative of it to test the composition and other specifications, e.g. microbiological counts, residue contents etc.
- On the basis of the tests the samples can be accepted or rejected. It is therefore very important that the samples taken are truly representative of the whole batch.

10.1 Laboratory items required

- Meat grinder with set of plates and knives
- Waring Blender
- Refrigerator
- Knives, drills and meat saw
- Glass jars with screw covers
- Spatulas of various sizes
- Sampling bottles, cups, containers

10.2 Acceptable sampling

- These are commonly used in the sampling of raw materials and finished products for acceptance.
- Acceptance sampling provides information on a particular lot to meet the desired quality assurance for obtaining raw material or finished goods.

10.3 Random sampling

- This is normally used in the sampling of meat and meat products.
- In this a limited number of units from the batch are sampled at random.
- It is important that the selection of the units to be sampled is truly random and not biased.

10.4 Sample labelling

- Whenever samples are taken they must be labelled.
- The label should be legible and stable to the sample container or package.
- The information required on the label should include.
  - Time and date of sampling
  - Identity of the supplier
  - Batch no.
  - Sample location

10.5 Precautions

- Label the sample completely for identification.
- Keep the sample refrigerated at all times even at the time of preparation and in transit.
- Grind through a meat grinder two or three times, mixing thoroughly each time.
- Grind and mix the sample rapidly and transfer to an air-tight container.
- Store in refrigerator and analyse as soon as possible.

❑❑❑

Chapter II

Analysis of Chemical Composition of Muscle Foods

Foods of animal origin, particularly muscle foods have wider market around the globe because they are rich source of proteins, lipids, vitamins and minerals, out of which, protein and lipids are considered to be the integral components of human diet. But amongst all meats poultry has some desirable properties over red meat that is excellent flavour, more tender meat, high protein and low fat content. Further, they are also efficient converters of feed in to animal protein of high biological value as compared to other livestock species. The other avian species, sometimes also called non-traditional poultry species namely duck, geese, guinea fowl, turkey and certain game birds (quail, pheasants, pigeon etc) are important in meat production. Although they represent a very small portion of total output in the present day, however, in the coming years, they may play a greater role to meet global protein demand. So, it is desired such valuable commodity should reach to the people with proper nutritional labelling with the confirmation of reliable tests.

1. Moisture

Water represents major constituents of muscle food. It ranges from 65-80% of total muscle. Water exists in the muscle in the bound, immobilised and free form. Of the total water, immobilised water (15%) retained in the space between myofillaments, while bound water (4-5%) attached with the protein molecules. Water held only by weak surface process is known as free water. Free water has important role in improving sensory quality of meat and can be easily determined by various methods, while bound water remain unaffected during processing of meat. Water serves as a medium for water soluble proteins, vitamins, glycogen, enzymes, hormones and other nutrients.

1.1 Preparation of sample

The meat samples subjected to moisture estimation should be free of bones, separable connective tissues, fat and fascia, and also be excised into fine pieces otherwise, thoroughly ground using meat grinder. The finely diced or ground meat samples are required to be stored in LDPE bags under chilled condition until further use.

1.2 Methods

Common methods used for determination of moisture are gravimetric method, thermogravimetric method, infrared absorption, microwave absorption and nuclear magnetic resonance (NMR).

1.2.1 Gravimetric method

1.2.1.1 Principle

The meat sample is dried at 100 ± 2°C for 16 hrs or until constant weight is obtained and the loss of moisture is recorded and calculated as percentage.

1.2.1.2 Requirements

Meat sample, hot air oven, desiccators, digital weighing balance, moisture cup, spatula, tissue paper roll etc.

1.2.1.3 Procedure

- Make moisture cup free of moisture in pre-heated hot air oven
- Transfer it to desiccators for cooling.
- Weigh the moisture cup with lid.
- Take 10g of finely ground composite meat sample into the moisture cup and weigh again.
- Place the weighed moisture cup into the pre-heated hot air oven at 100 ± 2°C for 16 hrs and cool in desiccators.
- Take the weight of the moisture cup and observe the moisture loss from the sample.
- Repeat the drying and cooling cycles until constant weight of the sample is achieved.

Calculation

$$\text{Moisture (\%)} = \frac{\text{(Wt. of sample + moisture cup before drying) - (Wt. of sample + moisture cup after drying)}}{\text{Wt. of sample}} \times 100$$

1.2.2 Thermogravimetric method

1.2.2.1 Principle

Thermogravimetric analysis (TGA) resembles an automated version of the standard oven-drying method, where moisture in a food is removed via heating using infrared lamp. The TGA instrumentation consists of a thermo-balance, which automatically measures and records the weight loss of a meat sample as a function of time and temperature while the sample is being heated.

1.2.2.2 Requirements

Meat sample, thermo balance equipped with infrared lamp, sample plate, spatula etc.

1.2.2.3 Procedure

- Since it is an automated method switch ON the equipment and open the lid by pressing the control button.
- Place about 5g of meat sample (less than <10g) onto the sample plate provided with the thermo balance.
- Cover the lid of the balance and press the run button and wait for 10-12 min until continuous beeps come.
- Percent moisture content reflects on the thermo balance indicating the moisture content of the sample.

1.2.3 Infrared absorption spectrometry

1.2.3.1 Principle

In this method IR beam passes through an optical filter, which consequently transmits energy at a specific wavelengths through the sample cell and then to a detector. The measuring spectral region of interest for determination of moisture or water is about 700-2400 nm since optimal absorption occurs at 1450 and 1940 nm wavelength are commonly used.

1.2.3.2 Requirements

Meat sample, infrared heater, sample tray, spatula etc.

1.2.3.3 Procedure

- Turn on the IR spectrum heater and calibrate using standards of known concentration and set the range of infrared spectrum.
- Keep sample onto the sample plate.
- Allow the infrared beams to pass through the sample and measure the maximum amount of absorption.
- Determine the moisture content in a sample by comparing the band intensity with that of the same band for standard concentrations of water.

1.2.4 Microwave absorption method

1.2.4.1 Principle

As water absorbs very high amount of microwave energy than a dry substance, it can be used to determine the moisture content of meat sample. The amount of water loss is determined by digital electronic weighing balance before and after drying and is calculated and expressed as percentage.

1.2.4.2 Requirements

Meat sample, microwave moisture meter consists of a constant source of microwave radiation, a wave guide, a detector, a microwave attenuator and amplifier, and an indicating meter.

1.2.4.3 Procedure

- Take two rectangular microwave resistant glass fiber pads on the digital weighing balance of microwave moisture analyzer chamber and 'tare'.
- Take out pads and keep about 5g of finely minced meat sample and distribute evenly onto the rough surface of one pad.
- Cover the sample with the second pad and place them together into the chamber.
- Expose the sample to microwave energy for 2-5 min at 100% power until constant weight of the sample is achieved.

- After completion of exposure time note the percent moisture from the panel.

1.2.5 Nuclear magnetic resonance

It is non-destructive method of moisture determination technique in which nuclear properties of protons is used to differentiate the proton NMR signal of water from the other hydrogen containing food substances with an accuracy of approximately 0.2 per cent.

1.2.6 Other methods

Mass spectrometer also use for determination of moisture content in muscle foods. Although mass spectrometry is widely utilized to identify unknown substances in food samples, the quantification of water is more problematic. The most significant problem is the "memory effect" where the previously analyzed sample influences the results of the following sample. Some success has been obtained by reacting cryogenically concentrated moisture with calcium carbide to yield acetylene, which is then quantified. However, mass spectrometry remains an uncommon method for moisture determination.

Notes:

- Moisture determination using TGA seems to give results similar to other methods. The water content of flour as measured by TGA was found to be comparable with that of the Karl Fischer method. The amount of residual moisture in glassy sugars after lyophilization and 1 week storage over P_2O_5 was similar whether determined by TGA, hot air oven, or vacuum oven. In addition to total moisture contents, TGA can also be used to quantify chemically bonded water of hydration.
- Since moisture is continuously evaporated from the sample, wait until sample has reached a constant weight or beeps. Keep some time interval for subsequent sample analysis to cool down and proper functioning of equipment. Care must be taken to avoid thermal decomposition of the sample which would lead to erroneous results.
- Calibration of the infrared spectrum should be done prior to use with the standards of known concentration.

2. Protein

Proteins are key component of all animal tissues. During protein formation amino acids are formed together in different array and exist as polypeptide chain, and thus as many as twenty different amino acids may form together in polypeptide chain. Thus all proteins differ from each other according to their functions, location in body, and also number and sequence of amino acids that make up the polypeptide backbone. As a result they have different molecular structures, nutritional attributes and physiochemical properties.

Nutritionally all proteins have important role as building block of body and other functions and as the source of essential amino-acids like lysine, tryptophan, methionine, leucine, isoleucine and valine. Since proteins are the major structural components of muscle foods they can influence tenderness of meat. Indeed, some purified proteins often used as texture modifying agents due to their ability to provide good gelling property, emulsification as well as foaming properties and thickeners. Some water soluble proteins, particularly enzymes which are capable of enhancing the rate of certain biochemical reactions to improve tenderness, flavour and other eating quality parameters. So, it is important to know the total proteins content in muscle foods and their nutritional importance, type and activity, functional properties etc to get fullest benefits for human health.

2.1 Crude protein

2.1.1 Micro-Kjeldahl method

2.1.1.1 Principle

Meat sample is digested in H_2SO_4 using $CuSO_4$, $5H_2O$ as catalyst. Anhydrous sodium sulphate (Na_2SO_4) or Na_2SO_4 elevate the boiling point and all the nitrogen compound of meat converted to ammonium sulphate. Subsequently the ammonium sulphate is hydrolysed by strong alkali (40% NaOH). By steam distillation the liberated ammonia is collected in boric acid solution containing "Toshiro's indicator". Ammonia with boric acid formed ammonium borate which is then titrated against standard H_2SO_4.

2.1.1.2 Requirements

- Equipments/apparatus: Kjeldahl flask, 250 mL volumetric flask, 50 mL burette, 100 mL conical flask, 5 or 10 mL pipette, digestion bench, micro-Kjeldahl distillation apparatus, glass beads and measuring cylinder 20 mL.

- Chemicals/reagents: Sulphuric acid (concentrated) AR, NaOH - 40%, digestion mixture (9.5 part sodium sulphate + 0.5 parts copper sulphate), standard H_2SO_4 - N/7 and Toshiro's indicator- (Methyl red-80 mg, Bromocresol green-20 mg and Methyl alcohol- 100 mL; add 10 ml of this solution to 1.0 Lit of 2% boric acid solution).

2.1.1.3 Procedure

- Weigh 2.0 g of meat in a butter/filter paper and transfer it to a Kjeldahl flask.
- Add 20 mL of concentrated H_2SO_4 and a pinch of digestion mixture (which will act as a catalyst).
- Digest the sample on digestion heater until the solution turns clear green.
- Transfer the digested sample into 250 mL volumetric flask with distilled water.
- Take 10 mL of aliquot into Micro-Kjeldahl distillation apparatus and add 20 mL of 40 % NaOH. Take 10 mL of Toshiro's indicator in a conical flask and dip the tip of silver tube into it.
- Heat the alkaline liquid by passing steam into it until boiling and keep it so till 30 mL of distillate is collected in the conical flask.
- Remove the conical flask after rinsing the tip with a little distilled water.
- Titrate the distillate with standard N/7 H_2SO_4 to a light pink endpoint.
- Always perform a blank test and correct the readings accordingly.

Calculation

$$\text{Protein (\%)} = \frac{\text{Amount of acid consumed (N/7 } H_2SO_4\text{) x 0.0002 x 250}}{\text{Weight of sample} \times \text{mL of aliquot taken}} \times 100 \text{x} 6.25$$

2.1.2 Kjeldahl method

2.1.2.1 Principle

When an organic matter is digested with concentrated H_2SO_4, organic nitrogen is converted into inorganic nitrogen or salt of nitrogen, say $(NH_4)_2SO_4$. The nitrogen in ammonical salt can be determined by distillation with an alkali in a Kjeldahl's apparatus. The solution of the salt is distilled with 40 per cent sodium hydroxide (NaOH) and ammonia (NH_3) thus liberated is absorbed in a known excess of 4 per cent boric acid solution. The amount of ammonia absorbed is determined by titration with standard acid ($N/_{10}$ HCl or H_2SO_4) using methyl red and Bromocresol green as indicator. The end point is indicated by the change of colour from blue to pink.

2.1.2.2 Apparatus

- Kjeldahl's digestion set
- Kjeldahl's distillation apparatus.
- Burette
- Pipette 2 mL, 10 mL
- Titration flask 100 mL

2.1.2.3 Reagents

- $N/_{10}$ Hydrochloric acid (HCl)
- 4% Boric acid: Dissolve approximately 40 gm of boric acid in 1 litre of distilled water. Add 5 ml of mixed indicator and adjust the stock solution by adding diluted HCl so that it takes slight pink colour.
- Mixed indicator: Take 0.5 g of Bromocresol green and 0.1 g of methyl red and dissolve in 100 ml of 95 per cent ethanol, adjust this solution with diluted NaOH or HCl to bluish purple colour.
- 40 per cent Sodium hydroxide (NaOH) – Dissolve approximately 400g of caustic soda (NaOH) in 1 litre of water.
- Digestion mixture: 10g potassium sulphate (K_2SO_4), 0.5g copper sulphate ($CuSO_4$) and 1 g of ferrous sulphate ($FeSO_4$) are mixed well. Here potassium sulphate acts by raising boiling point of H_2SO_4 and copper sulphate acts as catalyst to promote oxidation of protein in the sample.

2.1.2.4 Procedure

- Exactly weigh 0.5g of the sample and transfer to Kjeldahl's digestion flask (100 ml).
- Add 10 ml of concentrated H_2SO_4 to it and also mix drench of digestion mixture.
- Gently heat and then move strongly after frothing has ceased.
- Stop heating when the solution becomes clear or colourless.
- Cool to the room temperature.
- Dilute the solution with distilled water to make the volume 100 ml.
- Before starting the actual distillation, take blank reading to avoid any nitrogen retained in the apparatus.
- Pipette out 10 mL of 4 per cent boric acid solution into a 100 mL conical flask.
- Add 2 drops of mixed indicator to it and fit the conical flask to the distillation apparatus.
- Take 2 mL of digestion solution and put in the distillation apparatus.
- Add 5 mL of 40 per cent sodium hydroxide solution.
- Heat the distillation apparatus over the hot plate.
- Collect liberated ammonia in the boric acid keeping the tip dipped into it.
- Continue distillation till no more ammonia is coming then disconnect the burner.
- Take $^{N}/_{10}$ hydrochloric acid in the burette.
- Take the blank reading.
- Titrate the ammonia collected in the boric acid against the standard acid till the blue colour convert into pink colour.

Calculation

$$\text{Nitrogen (\%)} = \frac{0.0014 \times \text{Vol. of digested sample made} \times \text{Vol. of N/10 HCl used} \times 100}{\text{Wt. of sample taken} \times \text{Vol. of aliquot taken}} = \frac{0.0014 \times V1 \times V3 \times 100}{W \times V2}$$

Per cent crude protein = per cent Nitrogen x 6.25

Where 6.25 is the general factor.

2.1.3 Biuret method

2.1.3.1 Principle

Biuret reagent reacts with the peptide bonds of protein. There is formation of coordination complex between peptide bond of protein and cuprous ions of copper sulphate present in the biuret reagent. This complex is blue in colour and its absorbance is recorded at 540 nm in UV- spectrophotometer.

2.1.3.2 Apparatus and Chemicals

Test tubes, Pipettes, Beakers, Reagent bottle, Chemical balance, Spectrophotometer, Biuret reagent (in 1 Litre distilled water): KI- 2.5g, $CuSO_4$- 1.5g, Potassium sodium tartrate- 4.25g, NaOH- 4g

2.1.3.3 Procedure

- Standard BSA (Bovine Serum Albumin) having concentration of 10 mg/ml was used. In two test tubes No.1 and No.2 standard BSA 0.2 ml and buffalo serum three times diluted 0.2 ml were taken respectively. Distilled water 0.8 ml was added to both the test tubes to make 1 ml volume.
- In the test tube No.3, blank sample containing 1 ml distilled water was taken.
- 5 ml of Biuret reagent was added to each test tube i.e. No.1, 2 and 3.
- Blue colour was developed after 30 min. OD was recorded at 540 nm.
- Both standard and test sample were taken in duplicate.
- Calculation was made using the formula to know the protein concentration in the test sample.

Calculation

$$\text{Protein (gm/100ml)} = \frac{\text{O.D. test}}{\text{O. D. std}} \times \text{conc. of std (mg)} \times \frac{100}{\text{Vol taken}} \times \frac{1}{1000} \times \frac{1}{3}$$

Note:

1. This method is more selective, but less sensitive and gives colour when the concentration of protein is in mg range.

2.1.4 Lowry's method

2.1.4.1 Principle

This method combines the use of Biuret reaction of protein with Cu^{2+} ions in alkali and reduction of phosphomolybdic and phosphotungstic acid in Folin's reagent by the aromatic amino acids viz., tyrosine, tryptophan, phenylalanine present in the protein to produce a more intense coloured product which can be quantitatively estimated by spectrophotometer at 750nm.

The method has the advantage of applicability to dried material as well as the solutions and it is very sensitive. Sample contains as little as 5µg of protein can be readily analyzed. The basis of the assay is thought to be the production of cuprous ions which reduce the F-C reagent.

2.1.4.2 Apparatus and chemicals

- Test tubes, Pipettes, Beakers, Reagent bottle, Chemical balance, Spectrophotometer.
- Copper Reagent- 1% copper Sulphate solution- 0.5 mL, 2% Potassium sodium tartrate- 0.5 ml, 2% Na_2CO_3 in 0.1N NaOH- 50 mL.
- Folin's reagent: 1:1 diluted with distilled water (2N solution) or dilute 1 volume of commercial Folin's reagent with 1 volume of 0.1N NaOH.
- Protein standard solution Bovine serum albumin (1mg/mL).

2.1.4.3 Procedure

- In the test tubes numbered 1, 2, 3, 4, 5 and 6 standard protein solution 10 times diluted (i.e. 0.1mg/ml) was taken 0.25, 0.5, 0.75, 1.0, 1.5 and 2.0 mL to get a concentration of protein 25, 50, 75, 100, 150 and 200µg, respectively and in test tube No. 7, blank was taken and in the test tube No.8, 0.1 mL sample (unknown) was taken.

- The volume of each test tube was made up to 2 mL by using 0.1N NaOH. Then 2 mL of copper reagent was added to each test tube and waited for 10 min.
- Then 0.5 ml of Folin's reagent (1:1 dilution) was mixed into each test tube and waited for 30 min. O. D was recorded at 750nm.
- A standard curve was plotted using the protein concentration (μg) of standard solutions in X-axis and respective O.D. in Y-axis.
- Using this standard curve, the concentration of protein of unknown sample was estimated.

2.1.5 Bradford method (UV Spectroscopy method)

2.1.5.1 Principle

Bradford method is based on the observation that the absorbance maximum for an acidic solution of Coomassie Brilliant Blue G-250 (CBB) shifts from 465 nm to 595 nm when binding to protein occurs. Both hydrophobic and ionic interactions stabilize the anionic form of the dye, causing a visible colour change. The assay is useful since the extinction coefficient of a dye-albumin complex solution is constant over a 10-fold concentration range.

2.1.5.2 Apparatus and chemicals

- Spectrophotometer, cuvettes and 1 N NaOH
- Bradford reagent: Dissolve 100 mg Coomassie Brilliant Blue G-250 in 50 mL 95% ethanol; add 100 ml 85% (w/v) phosphoric acid. Dilute to 1 litre when the dye has completely dissolved, and filter through Whatman No. 1 filter paper just before use. The Bradford reagent should be a light brown in colour. Filtration may have to be repeated to rid the reagent of blue components. The Bio-Rad concentrate is expensive, but the lots of dye used have apparently been screened for maximum effectiveness. "Homemade" reagent works quite well but is usually not as sensitive as the Bio-Rad product.

2.1.5.3 Procedure

- Warm up the spectrophotometer before use.

- Dilute the sample so that protein concentration may range from 5-100 μg/ 100 μL.
- Add an equal volume of 1 M NaOH to each sample and vortex.
- Prepare standards containing a range of 5-100 micrograms protein (ovalbumin) in 100 μL volume.
- Add 5 ml dye reagent and incubate 5 min.
- Measure the absorbance at 595 nm.

Note:

1. Prepare a linear standard curve of absorbance vs. protein and determine amounts from the curve or using linear formula and express the protein amount in μg/g or mL.

2.2 Sarcoplasmic proteins

Muscle protein based on their solubility can be classified as water soluble proteins (sarcoplasmic), salt soluble proteins (myofibrillar) and acid soluble proteins (collagen, elastin, reticulin) with a percent proportion of 5, 11.5 and 2.5 % respectively out of total 19 %. The myofibrillar proteins play a vital role in meat processing as an emulsifier of fat and binder. During the storage of meat, amongst the proteins, the water soluble proteins are attacked by the proteolytic enzymes of bacteria while the structural proteins are the last to be proteolysed. The percent protein and the break down products are used as an indicator of extent of proteolysis during storage of meat.

2.2.1 Principle

The protein fractions are extracted in the suitable medium depending upon the maximum extractability and quantitation is done by estimating nitrogen by Kjeldahl method.

2.2.2 Apparatus and chemicals

Digestion flask, micro Kjeldahl apparatus, spectrophotometer and refrigerated centrifuge.

2.2.3 Procedure

- Weigh about 20 g meat in a centrifuge tube.

- Add 30 mL of chilled distilled water and blend in a tissue homogenizer for 2 min.
- Transfer the homogenate quantitatively to volumetric flask and make the volume to 200 mL.
- Keep overnight at 4°C and centrifuge at 3000 rpm for 15 min in refrigerated centrifuge.
- Measure nitrogen in the supernatant by micro Kjeldahl method as mentioned earlier.

2.3 Myofibrillar proteins

- Dispense the residue from above estimation in 200 mL of 0.67 M NaCl solution.
- Keep overnight at 4°C and centrifuge at 3000 rpm for 15 min.
- Measure nitrogen in the supernatant by micro Kjeldahl method.

2.4 Stromal proteins (Acid soluble protein)

- The residue obtained after extraction of myofibrillar proteins can be further processed for extraction of stromal proteins.
- For this first defat the residue by stirring in excess of acetone for 24 h at 4°C.
- Wash the residue in ether and the centrifuge.
- Homogenize the defatted residue with 10 mL of 0.5 M acetic acid and keep overnight at 0–4°C.
- Centrifuge it, collect the supernatant and label as acid extractable stromal proteins.
- Re-extract the residue by stirring in 10 mL of 0.1N sodium hydroxide at 95–98°C for 1 h.
- Keep overnight at 4°C.
- Centrifuge the content, collect the supernatant and label it as alkali extractable stromal proteins.
- Dry the insoluble protein fraction with acetone and ether, weigh and express as g per 100 g wet tissue.

2.5 Collagen (Hydoxyproline estimation)

The major component of connective tissue is collagen, which contains the amino acid L-hydroxyproline in much higher levels than found in the muscles. Hydroxyproline is a derived amino acid present only in connective tissue and higher in collagen (13 - 14 %). It is therefore, used as a measure of the connective tissue. It is formed by the hydroxylation of proline in the presence of ascorbic acid. Hydroxyproline concentration in beef muscles is reported to range between 200 - 770 µg/g. Although excessive proteolysis of the collagen and elastin of connective tissue might appear to be the most likely change causing increased tenderness, the portion of connective tissue is not normally changed during conditioning in skeletal muscle. This was evidenced by no increase in water soluble hydroxyproline, even after storage of sterile, fresh meat for one year at 37°C.

By measuring L-hydroxyproline content the connective tissue content of raw meat can be estimated. Collagen content of meat is determined by multiplying hydroxyproline content with 7.25.

2.5.1 Principle

Meat is hydrolyzed in a solution of HCl. The resultant hydroxyproline is oxidized with chromatin - T and reacted with 4 - dimethyl aminobenzaldehyde (DMEB). The red colour developed is measured photometrically.

2.5.2 Apparatus and chemicals

- Spectrophotometer, cuvette, Shaker
- HCl, NaOH, Proponol-1, Isopropyl alchohol (Propanol-2)
- Buffer solution (pH 6.0)-Dissolve 50 g of citric acid monohydrate, 12 mL acetic acid, 120 g sodium acetate trihydrate and 34 g of NaOH in distilled water and dilute to 1 litre.
- Oxidizing agent: Take 1.41 g of Chloramin-T, add 10 mL of water, 10 mL propanol-1 and 80 mL of above buffer. Mix this solution with 200 mL of water and 300 mL of propanol-1.
- Colour reagent: Add 65 mL of propanol- 2 to 35 mL of perchloric acid containing 10 g of 4-dimethyl aminobenzaldehyde (DMEB).

1.2.5.1 Procedure

- Weigh accurately 4 g of thoroughly mixed muscle sample and transfer to a boiling flask attached with a water cooled condenser.
- Add 100 mL 6N HCl and continue hydrolysis on a water bath for 6 – 8h.
- Filter the hot hydrolysate through a sintered glass funnel (G – 4), wash the flask three times with 6N HCl and add to filtrate as above.
- Dilute the hydrolysate up to 200 mL.
- Take 5 mL of the hydrolysate in a glass beaker and neutralize with 10 % NaOH initially, followed by 1N NaOH adjusting pH to 6.8.
- Make up the volume of the hydrolysate to 100 mL.
- Take 5 mL of hydrolysate in a test tube and add 2 mL of oxidizing reagent.
- Mix the contents on a shaker and keep at room temperature for 20 min.
- Add 2 mL of freshly prepared colour reagent and mix.
- Transfer the test tube to water bath (maintained at 60°C) for exactly 15 min.
- Cool the test tube under running water for at least 3 min and read the absorbance at 560 nm immediately in a spectrophotometer.
- Calculate the concentration from the regression equation computed from the reference values.

Calculation

$$\text{Hydroxyproline (mg/100 g)} = \frac{\text{OD of unknown} \times \text{Concentration of standard}}{\text{OD of standard}}$$

Collagen % (Net weight) = 7.25 × hydroxyproline (mg/100 g)

From calibration curve the calculation is given below

Hydroxyproline (%) = 5C/MV

C = concentration of diluted hydrolysate in μg/mL

M = weight of sample in g

V = volume of aliquot of hydrolysate taken for dilution in mL (usually 5 mL)

Collagen % (wet weight) = 7.25 × hydroxyproline (mg/100g)

Notes:

1. For reference values of hydroxyproline weigh accurately 100 mg of standard hydroxyproline in a 100 mL volumetric flask. Add little water and a drop of 6N HCl. Make the volume with distilled water. Store it (stock solution) at 4°C for further use.
2. For preparation of working standard, take appropriate amount of stock solution and make 5 serial dilutions in test tube using 0.5, 1.0, 1.5, 2.0 and 2.5μg/mL and follow the dilutions as described above adding oxidizing reagent and colouring agents. Read the colour at 560 nm for calculating regression equation.

3. Lipid analysis

Lipid or fat deposited in muscle has many functions. It improves delicacy of muscle foods by influencing flavour, juiciness and texture. However, the lipid profiles of meats from different animals vary considerably (1.5–13 %) and it depends on species, age, sex, plan of nutrition, processing etc. The major fat of animal tissues comprised of triglycerides or true fat. Other fatty deposits include mono and polyunsaturated fatty acids, phospholipids and cholesterol. But lipid has some deleterious effects on foods and also on human health. So, its determination is important.

Many organic solvents or combinations of solvent are used to extract lipids from muscle foods, but a suitable solvent should be non-toxic, has better extraction efficiency, economy and off-course should have no or little detrimental effects to the environment. However, choice of solvent may vary depending on the nature of food matrix and lipid components. In general, triglycerides (neutral lipid, true fat) are extracted by non-polar solvents such as petroleum ether, n-hexane or supercritical carbon dioxide while phospholipids and glycolipids (polar lipids) are extracted using polar solvents for quantitative determination, but care must be taken to avoid or at least minimize auto or enzymatic oxidation of polyunsaturated fatty acids.

3.1 Ether extracts (Soxhlet method)

3.1.1 Principle

The crude fat is extracted with petroleum ether from the dried sample. The solvent is removed by evaporation and the residue of fat is weighed and calculated.

3.1.2 Apparatus and chemicals

- Soxhlet's extraction apparatus, hot air oven, thimbles, weighing balance and desiccators.
- Petroleum ether (Boiling point 40-60°C or 60-80°C).

3.1.3 Procedure

- Set the Soxhlet's apparatus, take the weight of round bottom flask and gently pour 100 ml petroleum ether.
- Take about 2-3 g well ground dried sample in an extraction thimble and plug the open end of the thimble with absorbent cotton.
- Place the thimble in the extractor (the open end up) and connect with the round bottom flask. Connect the extractor to a reflux condenser.
- Extract the sample under reflux for 5-6 hours or 100 cycles of ether through the condenser.
- Evaporate the petroleum ether extract to dryness and add 2 ml acetone. Blow air gently into the flask to remove the last traces of solvent.
- Dry the flask containing the fat residue in a hot air oven at 100°C for 5 minutes. Cool in a desiccator and weight.

Calculations

Let weight (g) of sample before drying = W_1

Weight (g) of flask empty = W_2

Weight (g) of flask with fat = W_3

$$\text{Extractable Fat or crude fat (\%)} = \frac{W_3 - W_2}{W_1} \times 100$$

Or,

$$\text{Extractable Fat or crude fat (\%)} = \frac{\text{Weight of fat}}{\text{Weight sample}} \times 100$$

3.2 Total lipids (Gravimetric method)

3.2.1 Requirements

- Hot air oven, weighing balance, stainless steel planchet, aliquot of lipid extract etc

3.2.2 Procedure

- The total lipids of the samples were determined gravimetrically by a method described by Folch and Sloane-Stanley (1957).
- Take 1 mL of aliquot of the lipid extract into dried stainless steel planchets with constant predetrmined weights.
- The samples were dried at 60°C in a hot air oven to a constant weight.
- Total lipids were expressed as mg/g of a sample.

3.3 Total phospholipids

3.3.1 Principle

Total phospholipids were estimated by determining the phosphorus content of the lipid extract by converting into inorganic phosphorus. The modified method of Marinetti (1962) is used for the estimation of phosphorus.

3.3.2 Apparatus and reagents

- Micropipette, spectrophotometer, hot water bath, digestion bench, measuring cylinder.
- Lipid extract, potassium dihydrogen phosphate, distilled water, ammonium molybdate and ANSA (1 Amino 2- Naphthol 4 Sulfonic acid).

- *Standard phosphorus solution*: Dissolve 0.35 g of potassium dihydrogen phosphate (KH_2PO_4) in 10 mL of 10 N H_2SO_4 and finally make volume upto 1Lit using distilled water. This contains 0.4 mg of phosphorous/5 mL.
- *Ammonium molybdate solution*: Dissolve 25 g of ammonium molybdate in 200 ml of distilled water. Add 300 mLof 10 N H_2SO_4. Make up to 1 lit using distilled water.
- ANSA (1 Amino 2- Naphthol 4 Sulfonic acid): Dissolve 0.5 g of aminonaphthol sulphonic acid in 200 mL of 15 percent anhydrous sodium bisulphite followed by addition of 1 g of anhydrous sodium sulphite. The reagent is stable for one week in amber colour bottle under 4°C.

3.3.3 Procedure

- Take accurately 25 µL of lipid extract (make volume up to 5 mL with chloroform), standard phosphate solution (50 µl) containing 0.4 mg/5 mL phosphorous separately in a test tube.
- Evaporate the tubes to dryness and add 1 mL of 60 % perchloric acid for digestion in over dry water bath for 15 min.
- After digestion, add 0.5 mL of 2.5 % ammonium molybdate solution followed by 0.2 ml of ANSA reagent (1 Amino 2- Naphthol 4 Sulfonic acid).
- Mix well and add 7.0 mL of distilled water.
- Heat the tubes in water bath at 55 - 60°C for 7 min and cool to room temperature.
- Read blue colour at 620 nm in spectrophotometer.
- Calculate phospholipid content by multiplying inorganic phosphorus content with a factor of 25 and express as mg/g of sample.
- Prepare blank with perchloric acid only and treat in a similar manner.

Calculation

$$\text{Phosphorous (mg/g)} = \frac{\text{OD of unknown} \times \text{conc. of std.} \times \text{volume of lipid sample} \times 1}{\text{OD of std} \times \text{vol use for estimation} \times \text{wt of sample} \times 1000}$$

$$\text{Phospholipid (mg/g)} = 25 \times \text{phosphorous (mg/g)}$$

3.4 Total cholesterol

Though the consequences of dietary cholesterol on human health are ambiguous, it is important to determine total cholesterol content in all foods of animal origin. Cholesterol occurs in minute quantity and retain in muscle tissue either as free or esterified forms in combination with fatty acids. Meats from most food animals contain total cholesterol in the range of 55-70 mg/100 g while egg and offal contain total cholesterol in the range of 460- 800 mg/100 g and 1000-12000 mg/100 g, respectively. Total cholesterol in the lipid extracts were determined by adopting the method described by Hanel and dam (1955).

Method I (Acetyl chloride method)

3.4.1 Principle

The cholesterol reacts with the $ZnCl_2$ in the presence of acetyl chloride and heat and form pinkish red colour compound which is measured spectrophotometrically.

3.4.2 Apparatus and chemicals

- Spectrophotometer, Micro pipette, Water bath and Measuring cylinder.
- Lipid extract, Chloroform, $ZnCl_2$ reagent (Dissolve 40 g anhydrous $ZnCl_2$ in 150 mL glacial acetic acid at 80°C for 2.5 h and filter through glass wool), Acetyl chloride and Standard cholesterol (1 mg/mL in Chloroform)

3.4.3 Procedure

- Accurately measure 100 μL of lipid extract (volume make up to 5 mL with chloroform) and standard cholesterol separately in a test tube and evaporate to dryness.
- Add 2 mL of chloroform, 1 mL $ZnCl_2$ reagent and 1 mL acetyl chloride.
- Heat in water bath at 50°C for 10 min.
- For blank use 2 mL chloroform, 1 mL each of $ZnCl_2$ reagent and acetyl chloride.
- Read the optical density (pinkish red colour) at 528 nm in a spectrophotometer.

Calculation

$$\text{Cholesterol (mg/100 g)} = \frac{\text{OD unknown}}{\text{OD standard}} \times \frac{\text{Conc. Std} \times 5}{0.05} \times \frac{100}{1 \times 1000}$$

Method II

3.4.4 Principle

The cholesterol react with the $ZnCl_2$ in the presence of acetyl chloride and heat and form pinkish red colour compound which is measured spectrophotometrically.

3.4.5 Apparatus and chemicals

- Spectrophotometer, Micropipette, Water bath and Measuring cylinder
- Lipid extract
- Chloroform
- Glacial acetic acid
- Concentrate sulphuric acid
- $FeCl_3$- H_2SO_4 reagent: Dissolve 10 g of $FeCl_3$ in 100 mL acetic acid. Then 1 mL of $FeCl_3$ solution diluted to 100 mL with concentrated H_2SO_4.
- Standard cholesterol: 1 mg/mL in Chloroform

3.4.6 Procedure

- Take 250 μL of lipid extract (make volume upto 5 mL with chloroform) and 50 μl standard solution of cholesterol (1 mg/ mL) separately in test tubes and kept in water bath 55-66°C to evaporate chloroform.
- Add 3 ml of acetic acid in dried test tubes.
- Add 0.1 mL distilled water and 2 mL $FeCl_3$- H_2SO_4 reagent.
- Mix well and keep for half hour to develop colour.
- Prepare the blank with acetic acid only and treated in a similar fashion.
- Measure the optical density at 560 nm in a spectrophotometer and express as mg/g of tissues.

Calculation

$$\text{Cholesterol (mg/100 g)} = \frac{\text{OD unknown}}{\text{OD standard}} \times \frac{\text{Conc. Std} \times 5}{0.25 \times 2 \times 10 \times 1000}$$

3.5 Fatty acid profile (GLC method)

Gas chromatography still remains as the most valuable and efficient method of resolution and quantitation of fatty acids. This technique is based on the separation of short chain fatty acids in the free form. But these compounds require exhaustive pre-treatment for their separation and detection. Since the instrumentation has become more and more sophisticated with the development of new detectors, new columns, new injectors, and new ovens this technique became easier.

3.5.1 Principle

The lipid extract is converted into methyl/acyl esters and run into the GLC along with the standards and compared on the basis of retention time at the standard conditions.

3.5.2 Apparatus and chemicals

- Gas Liquid Chromatography with Flame Ionization Detector (FID), Columns packed with 20% diethylene glycol adipate (DEGA) on 101 chromosorb (60-80 mesh), Separating funnel, Pipettes, Funnels, Filter paper, Measuring cylinder, Micropipette, Vacuum Rotary Evaporator.
- 10% alcoholic KOH, HCl, Hexane, Distilled water, carrier gas etc

3.5.3 Procedure

- Take 2 μL of the sample extract and inject using a microsyringe (Hamilton, Reno, NV) in GLC equipped with flame ionization detector fitted with 6 % butane-diol-succinate on chromosorb WAW-DWCS column 6 feet in length and 1/4 inches in outer diameter.
- Set the equipment for the separation of compounds at oven temperature: 190–200°C, injector temperature: 250°C, detector

temperature: 250°C, hydrogen flow: 40 ml/min, nitrogen flow: 60 ml/min and air flow: 300–400 ml/min.

- Identify the peaks on comparison of their retention time with the standard fatty acyl esters.
- Calculate the relative concentration of fatty acids automatically by data jet integrator 5700.

3.6 Iodine value

3.6.1 Principle

The unsaturated fatty acids have the ability to absorb a definite quantity of iodine when reacted with iodine chloride or iodine bromide to form saturated compounds. The grams of iodine absorbed by 100 gram of fat is a measure of the un-saturation of fat and is expressed as the iodine value

3.6.2 Reagents

- Chloroform reagent AR.
- 15 % potassium iodide in volumetric flask with freshly boiled and cooled distilled water.
- Iodine bromide solution- Dissolve 13.615 g pure iodine in 825 ml of glacial acetic acid, cool and add 3 ml of bromine solution.
- Sodium thiosulphate 0.1N ($Na_2S_2O_3$).
- Starch indicator for titration.

3.6.3 Procedure

- Weigh 0.5 g of fat in iodine flask and add 10 ml of chloroform. Shake until fat is dissolved.
- Add 25 ml of iodine solution and allow to stand for 30 minutes with occasional shaking.
- Add 10 ml of 15% KI and shake.
- Add 100 ml of boiled and cooled distilled water.
- Titrate with 0.1 $Na_2S_2O_3$. As yellow colour becomes faint add few drops of starch indicator and titrate till the blue colour of top layer disappears.

Calculation

Iodine/10 g of fat = A x N of $Na_2S_2O_3$ x 126.91/weight of sample

A = ml of $Na_2S_2O_3$ required for blank – ml of $Na_2S_2O_3$ required for sample

3.7 Saponification number

3.7.1 Principle

Saponification is reaction between carboxylic group of fatty acids and alkali. It is defined as the mili grams of KOH required to saponify one gram of fat. It indicates about the chain length of fatty acids in a fat. If the chain length is more there will be less number of fatty acids or carboxylic group available for saponification in given quantity of fat, hence, will have less saponification number.

3.7.2 Reagents

- 0.5 N HCl
- 1 % Phenolphthalein solution in 95% alcohol.
- KOH solution: 35 to 40 g of KOH pellets are dissolved in 20 ml of water to which alcohol (95%) is added to make 1liter. The solution is allowed to settle overnight and the supernatant is used.

3.7.3 Procedure

- Weigh about 2 g of sample accurately in a 250 ml round bottom flask.
- Add 25 ml of alcoholic KOH solution and heat the flask in boiling water bath for 1 hour.
- Add 1 ml of phenolphthalein solution and titrate the excess alkali against 0.5 N HCl.
- Repeat above without the oil or fat to obtain the blank value (b).

Calculation

- Following equation is used to calculate the saponification number.

$$\text{Saponification number} = \frac{(b - a) \times 0.02805 \times 1000}{\text{Weight in g of substance}}$$

Note:

1. 1 ml of 0.5 N HCl is equivalent to 0.02805 g of KOH.

4. Crude fibre

4.1 Principle

A fat free sample is treated with boiling sulphuric acid and subsequently boiling in sodium hydroxide. The residue after subtraction of the ash is regarded as fibre.

4.2 Apparatus and chemicals

- Glass Beakers, Bunchner funnel, Muffle furnance, Crucibles, Weighing balance, Desiccators and Water bath.
- Hydrochloric acid (1% v/v),
- Sulphuric acid stock solution 10 % w/v (55 ml conc. H_2SO_4 diluted to 1 litre),
- Sulphuric acid working solution 1.25% (125 mL of stock solution diluted to 1 litre),
- Sodium hydroxide stock solution 10% w/v (100gm NaOH in 1 litre DW),
- Sodium hydroxide working solution 1.25% (125 ml of stock solution diluted to 1 litre),
- Antifoam : 2% Silicon antifoam in CCl_4.

4.3 Procedure

- Weigh (1-2g) of fat free dried sample in a 1 litre beaker.
- Add 200 mL 1.25% (hot) H_2SO_4 and few drops of antifoam.
- Heat to boiling within 1 minute on the crude fibre apparatus.
- Boil the solution exactly for 30 minutes under bulb condensers. Rotate the beaker occasionally to mix the contents and remove the particles from the side.
- Filter the contents of the beaker through Bunchner funnel.

- Wash the sample back into the tall beaker with 200 mL 1.25% sodium hydroxide.
- Boil for exactly 30 minutes.
- Transfer all insoluble matter to the sintered crucible by means of boiling water till acid free.
- Wash twice with alcohol.
- Wash three times with acetone.
- Dry at 100°C to constant weight.
- Ash in a muffle furnace at 550°C for 1 hour.
- Cool crucible in a desiccators and reweigh.

Calculation

Let weight (g) of sample = W_1

Weight (g) of insoluble matter = W_2

Weight (g) of Ash = W_3

$$\text{The fibre (\%)} = \frac{W_2 - W_3}{W_1} \times 100$$

5. Mineral determination

The term "ash" refers to the inorganic residue remaining after total incineration of organic matter. The ash content is determined from the loss of weight, which occurs from complete oxidation of the sample at a high temperature (usually 500-600°C) through combustion and volatilization of organic materials. The ash obtained does not typically contain exactly the same type of minerals as those present in the original food because they are typically converted into a different molecular structure, such as oxides, phosphates, and sulphates. Some minerals may also be lost due to volatilization.

To ash a sample completely, heating continues until the resulting ash is uniform in colour, most commonly white or gray and free from particles of unburned organic material. Ashing may be accomplished by incineration over an open flame, in a muffle furnace, in a closed system in the presence of oxygen, by wet oxidation in the presence of sulphuric, nitric, and perchloric acids alone or in mixtures, or by microwave digestion.

The analysis of ash is important for several reasons. The ash content can be regarded as a general indicator of product quality. Ash analysis can also be used to determine food adulteration. Abnormally high ash content suggests the presence of an inorganic adulterant, such as sand or dirt, which could be further evaluated by determining acid-insoluble ash. Total ash content may be used to indicate the nutritional value of food products. More precise nutritional information is obtained by performing elemental analysis on the resulting ash.

5.1 Methods of ashing

The two primary ashing procedures are dry ashing and wet ashing, which are eventually utilized to determine the mineral content of the food. In dry ashing, the organic matter of the sample is oxidized by complete incineration at a high temperature in the presence of oxygen, whereas, in wet ashing the sample is oxidized with a mixture of concentrated strong acids. A more recent development in ashing methodologies is the use of microwaves to increase the speed of sample digestion. In addition to these direct methods, there are indirect techniques for determining specific ash components in foods, such as conductometric methods for measuring their total electrolyte contents. The selection of an ashing methodology depends on the purpose for which the ash is prepared, the minerals to be analyzed, and the method of analysis to be used.

5.1.1 Dry ashing

5.1.1.1 Principle

Dry ashing is the most standard method for determining the ash content of a food sample. The sample is commonly ignited at 550-600°C to oxidize all organic materials without flaming. The inorganic residue, which does not volatilize at that temperature, is called ash. Detailed dry ashing methodologies for specific food products can be found in the Official Methods of Analysis of AOAC International.

5.1.1.2 Apparatus and chemicals

- Muffle furnace (electric), thermostatically controlled Porcelain crucibles with lids, Analytical balance (0.1 mg sensitivity), Desiccators, Tongs, Marking ink (permanent type for crucibles), Bunsen burner, Hot-plate (thermostatically controlled), Tripod (iron), Steam bath, Atmospheric oven, Wash bottle, Double deionized water.

5.1.1.3 Procedure

- Place clean and labeled crucibles in a muffle furnace at 600°C for 1 h.
- Turn off the furnace and transfer partially cooled crucibles into a desiccators and cool to room temperature.
- Weigh crucibles quickly to prevent possible moisture absorption. Use metal tongs to move the crucibles after they are heated or dried (crucible preparation).
- Weigh accurately 2 g of dry food or 10 g of wet sample into the prepared pre-weighed crucible.
- For wet samples, dry the sample on a hot-plate or steam bath or in an atmospheric oven at 100°C for 1 h.
- Place the crucible on an iron tripod over a Bunsen burner or hot-plate and slowly char for about 30 min (under the hood). Heat cautiously to prevent excessive foaming and spattering. A few drops of olive oil can be added to reduce spattering. Omit this step for samples not rich in carbohydrates.
- Place the crucibles in muffle furnace set at 550°C for 12-18 h. Burn off the organic material until the samples become completely free from carbon and appear as light gray or white ash.
- If black carbon spots persist in the crucible due to incomplete oxidation of the samples, turn off the furnace, allow the sample to cool, add a few drops of concentrated nitric acid directly on to the unburnt spots, and switch on the furnace again. Raise the temperature to 600°C and leave 1-2 h depending on the incompleteness of the ashing.
- Turn off oven and allow it to cool. Opening a hot oven will cause ash to blow out of crucibles. Upon opening the cooled oven, cover crucibles with a lid or watch glass to prevent ash from blowing away.
- Transfer the partially cooled crucibles into a desiccator and continue cooling to room temperature. When cooled, weigh the crucible as quickly as possible to prevent moisture absorption.
- Save the ash sample if elemental analysis is to be performed.

Calculations

$$\%Ash = \frac{\text{Weight of residue x 100}}{\text{Sample wight}}$$

5.1.2 Wet ashing

For samples that are to undergo elemental analysis, wet ashing is more advantageous than dry ashing. The wet ashing method is preferable to the dry ashing procedure for digesting organic matter prior to the determination of mineral constituents because it eliminates difficulties resulting from losses of more volatile inorganic constituents during dry ashing and slow dissolution of the residue after dry ashing.

Although using a single acid is desirable, it is often not practical for the complete digestion of the sample Nitric acid functions as a good oxidant, but typically volatilizes before the sample is completely oxidized. Sulphuric acid aids in the digestion, but using perchloric acid with nitric acid greatly facilitates decomposition of many hard-to-digest organic compounds. However, great care must be taken when using perchloric acid because it can be explosive.

5.1.2.1 Principle

Wet ashing commonly employs concentrated nitric and perchloric acids to oxidize the organic matter of the food sample. These acids are partially removed by volatilization and the soluble mineral constituents remain dissolved in nitric acid. Any silica present is dehydrated and made insoluble.

5.1.2.2 Apparatus and chemicals

- Fume hood, constructed for safe exhaustion of perchloric acid and nitric acid fumes, Hot-plate (thermostatically controlled), Glassware (250mL beaker, 100 ml volumetric flask, Pyrex or similar quality), Watch glass, Goggles (protective glasses), Glass rod (for sample stirring and transfer), Glass boiling beads, Air oven, Steam bath.
- Nitric acid (69-71% concentrated), Perchloric acid (60-62% concentrated), Digestion acid (add 1 volume perchloric acid to 4 volumes nitric acid), Hydrochloric acid (approximately 2 M; add 1 volume hydrochloric acid (36% HCl) to 5 volumes deionized water).

5.1.2.3 Procedure

- Weigh accurately 1-2 g dry, ground sample into a 250 mL beaker. While wearing safety goggles, add 20 ml digestion acid and three boiling beads to the beaker under a fume hood.
- After addition of the digestion acid, allow the reaction to proceed in the hood at room temperature for 3-4 h with occasional swirling using hands and a glass rod, or leave overnight.
- Place the sample beaker on a hot-plate maintained at a temperature such that the liquid in the beaker just simmers. When the initial reaction has subsided, slowly increase the temperature of the hot plate to 350°C.
- Evaporate the digestion acid until dense white fumes are formed within the beaker. Cover the beaker with a watch glass.
- Continue the digestion until the fluid in the beaker becomes clear and no visible particles remain. If the solution darkens when the volume is reduced, remove the flask from the hot-plate, add 1 or 2 ml nitric acid and continue the digestion with occasional swirling.
- Remove the beaker from the hot-plate. Rinse the watch glass with deionized distilled water. Transfer the solution quantitatively to a 100 mL volumetric flask with deionized distilled water.
- Stopper the flask, thoroughly mix the solution and leave overnight. The water-insoluble and acid-insoluble silica will settle to the bottom and aliquots of the solution are drawn from the top, filtered, and stored in small polyethylene bottles for later analyses.
- The sample solution prepared can be used for the determination of various macro and trace minerals by atomic absorption spectrophotometry or other suitable method.

References

AOAC (1985). *Journal of AOAC* 68: 876.

Bendall, J.R. 1967. *Journal of Food and Agriculture* 18: 553–558.

Bradford, MM.1976. *Analytical Biochemistry 72:* 248-254.

British Pharmacopoeia Appendix X - C, p. 1057 (1963). A.O.A.C. Official method Cd 3-25.

Hanel HK, Dam H 1955. *Acta Chem Scandinivian* 9: 677-682.

Kang, C. K. and Rice E. E. 1970. *Journal of Food Science* 35: 563-565.

Koniecko, E.K. (1979) In Hand book for Meat Chemists, pp 68-69, Avery Publishing Group, New Jersey, USA.

Marinetti, G.V.J. 1962. *Lipid Research* 3: 1-20.

Narayanan, A.S. and Page, R.C. 1976. *Biol. Chemistry* 251: 1125-1130.

Prasad, R.L. and Singh, L. N. 1990. *Indian J. Meat Sci. Technol* 3(1): 22-28.

Stegman, H and Stadler, K. Clin.1967. *Chem. Acta* 18: 167.

Stoscheck, CM.1990 *Methods in Enzymology 182:* 50-69.

Woessner, J. F. 1961. *Arch. Biochem. Biophysics* 93: 440-447.

❑❑❑

Chapter III

Evaluation of Functional Quality of Meat

1. Water holding capacity (WHC)

Water holding capacity (WHC) is the ability of meat to retain its water with the application of external force such as cutting, grinding, pressing, heating etc. Water holding capacity of muscle tissue has a direct effect on shrinkage of meat during storage. WHC is especially critical in meat products manufacture that is prepared by combination of heating, grinding etc. Generally WHC is measured by two methods viz. Centrifugal method and Press method. WHC is affected by several factors which cause differentiation in muscles, such as species, age and the muscular function. It is found that WHC of pork is higher than that of beef. Although the age of the animals does not appear to be an influence with pork, meat from calves having greater WHC than adult cattle beef. These differences are further reflection of differences in the rate and extent of pH fall, the ultimate pH in pork and veal tending to be higher than that in cattle. Muscles having higher content of intramuscular fat tend to have a high water holding capacity.

1.1 Centrifugal method

1.1.1 Apparatus, chemicals and raw materials

- Minced meat sample, mechanical shaker, centrifuge tubes, measuring cylinders, glass rod, 0.6 M NaCl solution, refrigerated centrifuge machine, weighing balance etc

1.1.2 Procedure

- Take 20 g of finely minced meat sample in a centrifuge tube, add 30 mL of 0.6 M NaCl and mix with glass rod for 2 min.

- Hold the tube for 15 min at 4°C, shake for 1 min on a mechanical shaker and then centrifuge at 5,000 rpm for 10 min.
- Decant the supernatant in a measuring cylinder and note the volume.
- WHC is expressed as percentage.

Calculations

$$\text{WHC (\%)} = \frac{\text{Final volume - Initial volume}}{20} \times 100$$

1.2 Filter paper press method

1.2.1 Requirements

- Weighing balance, meat sample, glass plates or polythene sheets, weights (18.5 kg) and Whatman filter paper No. 1.

1.2.2 Procedure

- Take weight of two filter papers and then place exactly 0.5 g of finely minced meat sample at the centre in between the filter papers.
- Place polyethylene sheets or glass plates below and above filter papers on a flat surface.
- Apply pressure of 2.8 kg on it for 5 minutes.
- Remove the weights and weigh the meat flakes.
- Let dry the filter papers at room temperature and weigh.

Calculations

$$\text{Water Holding Capacity (\%)} = \frac{\text{Weight of meat flake}}{\text{Sample weight}} \times 100$$

2. Muscle fibre diameter (Microscopic method)

The essential structural unit of all muscles is the fibre. The fibres are long, narrow, multinucleated cells, which may stretch from one end to another end and may attain a length of 34 cm, although they are only 10-100 μ in diameter. In healthy animals the muscle fibre diameter differs from muscle to muscle, between species, breeds and sexes. Diameter is increased by age, plane of nutrition, training, by degree of post natal development in the body weight rather than body weight itself and by estradiol administration. The rate of increase in size of the muscle fibres declines as an animal approaches maturity. Muscle fibres of male are usually larger than those of female or castrates while those of male castrates being intermediate in fibre size.

As the animal grows older the total number of muscle fibres will decrease and remaining fibres will become larger. Thus, skeletal muscles in old age contain fewer fibres, which are larger than those at maturity.

2.1 Method I (Jermiah and Martin, 1977)

2.1.1 Apparatus and chemicals

- Tissue homogenizer, microscope, micrometer, cover slip, glass slide sucrose, EDTA

2.1.2 Procedure

- Weigh about 5 g of breast muscle from cross sectional surface sample.
- Cut into small cubes and homogenize twice for 15 sec at low speed with 5 sec interval in a solution containing 0.25 M sucrose and 1 mM EDTA to produce slurry.
- Transfer one or more drops of the slurry on to a glass slide and cover with a cover slip.
- Examine the suspension directly under a light microscope using a calibrated micrometer.
- Measure the muscle fibre diameter as the mean cross-sectional distance in micrometer between the external borders of the 20 randomly selected muscle fibres.

Method II (Formalin fixing method) (Tuma et al., 1962)

2.1.3 Apparatus and chemicals

- Tissue homogenizer, compound microscope, stage and ocular micrometer and 10 % formal saline.

2.1.4 Procedure

- Fix 1 inch muscle cube in 10 % formal saline for 24 h.
- Homogenize the tissue in waring blender at slow speed for 30 sec in 10 % formal saline so as to tease the muscle fibre.
- Use the compound microscope to measure the muscle fibre diameter using eye piece 10X and objective lens of 10X magnification.
- Calibrate the ocular micrometer by using stage micrometer, to know value of each digit in micron.
- Measure the diameter of each fibre at three different locations viz., two ends and middle portion.
- At least 50 straight fibres should be measured. Eliminate those fibres, which are wavy.
- Take average values and express the diameter in microns.

3. Measurement of sarcomere length (Microscopic method)

3.1 Principle

The unit of the myofibril between two adjacent Z – lines is called sarcomere. The sarcomere is the repeating structural unit of the myofibril and it is also basic unit in which the events of the muscle contraction relaxation cycle occur. Sarcomere length is not constant and its dimensions as well as those of I – band are dependent on the state of contraction at the time muscle is examined. In mammalian muscle at rest, a sarcomere length of 2.5 μm is rather typical. Sarcomere length is affected by conditioning, cooking, post-mortem temperature and mode of suspension of carcasses. Sarcomere length can be used for prediction of both longitudinal growth potential of muscle and as an indicator of meat tenderness during its conversion to meat.

3.2 Apparatus and chemicals

- Homogenizer, Light microscope with ocular micrometer, Glass slide etc.
- Sucrose solution

3.3 Procedure

- Weigh accurately 5 g of muscle from cross-sectional surface sample.
- Cut into small cubes and homogenize in a tissue homogenizer twice for 15 sec at low speed in 30 mL of 0.25 M sucrose solution for 60 sec.
- Transfer a drop of homogenate on to a glass slide and examine under a light microscope under oil immersion objective.
- If the fibres are not sufficiently broken apart, homogenize the sample for an additional period of 20-30 sec.
- Measure the sarcomere length using a calibrated ocular micrometer.
- Measure the sarcomere length of twenty myofibrils randomly.
- Calculate the average of sarcomere length and express in micrometer.

4. Myofibrillar fragmentation index (MFI)

Myofibrillar fragmentation Index (MFI) is related to the degradation of myofibrillar proteins during post-mortem storage of meat. A potential practical application of MFI would be to predict the level of tenderness in fresh and cooked steaks. The MFI values coincide with Waner Bratzler shear force values, sensory values and microscopic examination of muscle fibres. The MFI increases during refrigerated storage of muscle. It has been reported that MFI accounted for more than 50 % of the variation in loin steak tenderness and that MFI is more important indicator of tenderness in loin steak than collagen solubility or sarcomere length.

4.1 Method I (Phosphate-EDTA method, Oslon et al., 1976)

4.1.1 Apparatus and chemicals

- Isolating medium: 100 mM KCl, 20 mM potassium phosphate dibasic, 1 mM EDTA, 1 mM $MgCl_2$ and 1 mM Sodium azide dissolved in 1000 mL distilled water.
- Biuret reagent: Weigh 6 g sodium potassium tartrate and 1.5 g CuSO4, to this add 300 mL of 10 % NaOH with constant stirring. Dilute to 1000 mL with distilled water.

4.1.2 Procedure

- Take 4 g of minced meat and homogenized with 40 mL chilled isolating solution for 30 min.
- Centrifuge at 5000 rpm for 15 min and decant the supernatant.
- Re-suspend the sediment in 40 mL of isolating medium by using a stirring rod.
- Centrifuge again as above and decant the supernatant.
- Re-suspend the sediment in 10 mL of isolating medium, and filtered through polyethylene strainer to remove connective tissue and debris.
- Wash the strain with another 10 mL of isolating medium to facilitate passage of myofibrils through the strainer.
- Determine the protein concentration in the filtrate by **Biuret method.**

Calculation

$$MFI = OD \times 200$$

Note:

1. Adjust the protein concentration of the extract to 0.5 mg/mL by diluting with isolating medium to determine the protein concentration by Biuret method. Dilute the myofibril suspension and pour it into cuvette. Measure the optical density at 540 nm.

Method II (Sucrose – KCl method, Davis et al., 1980)

4.1.3 Apparatus and chemicals

- High speed tissue homozenizer, deep freezer, Weighing balance, Hot air oven, etc.
- Sucrose, Potassium chloride, Distilled water, Whatman filter paper No. 1 etc.

4.1.4

- Freeze the muscle cubes in an appropriate freezer.

- Weigh 10 g of frozen breast muscle cubes and transfer to a 250 mL centrifuge tube.
- Add 50 mL of cold solution of 0.25 M sucrose and 0.02 M potassium chloride.
- Thaw the muscle cube for 5 min.
- Homogenize the muscle cube in homogenizer for 40 sec at 45, 000 rpm with rat root rotor shaft aligned and positioned 1 mm below the surface of the solution.
- Filter the homogenate through a pre-weighed 250 μm stainless steel wire cloth screen in filtration unit stirring with a glass rod to expedite the filtration process.
- Blot the residue on a Whatman No 1 filter paper.
- Weigh the residue after 40 min of drying in a hot air oven at 40°C.
- Calculate the fragmentation index by multiplying the weight of the fraction remaining on the screen in g by 100.

5. Emulsion stability (ES)

5.1 Principle

Emulsion stability gives a rough idea about expected yield and quality, particularly texture and juiciness of finished emulsion based meat products.

5.2 Apparatus and chemicals/solvents

- Water bath, LDPE pouches, blotter/tissue paper, digital weighing balance etc.
- Distilled water.

5.3 Procedure

- Take about 20 g of meat emulsion and make into a round ball.
- Place it into a pre-weighed LDPE pouches and take the weight. Note down the weight of meat ball.
- Keep the sample with pouch into the preheated water bath (80°C) and hold at this temperature for 35 min.

- Remove the pouch and cool the sample.
- Weep out the juices with blotters/tissue paper and take weight of meat ball.
- Take at least three meat balls for each experiment.

Calculation

$$\text{Emulsion stability } (\%) = \frac{\text{Weight of meat balls after cooking}}{\text{Weight of raw meat balls}} \times 100$$

6. Emulsifying capacity (Swift et al., 1961)

6.1 Principle

Emulsifying capacity (EC) is the ability of proteins to emulsify or hold a maximum amount of fat under specific conditions. The emulsifying capacity and pH are highly correlated. Adjustment of pH of post-rigor poultry muscle to that of pre-rigor state restored the original high EC of pre-rigor muscle. The EC of meat proteins in the descending order is actin, myosin, actomyosin, sarcoplasmic proteins has been reported. The EC is minimum at iso-electric point of muscle proteins and increases on either side of pH. The EC is also influenced by the concentration of the salt soluble proteins, temperature, speed of mixing, bacterial load etc.

6.2 Apparatus and chemicals/solvents

- Analytical balance, high speed blender (15000 rpm)
- Sodium chloride, Distilled water, Refined vegetable oil etc

6.3 Procedure

- Weigh about 25 g of minced meat sample.
- Add 100 mL of 1M NaCl and keep overnight at 4°C.
- Homogenize at 13000 rpm to prepare the slurry.
- Weigh 2.5 g of slurry and add 37.5 mL of 1M NaCl and mix well.
- Initially add 50 mL refined edible oil and blend in a plastic emulsifying jar at 13000 rpm, simultaneously running down measured quantity of oil @ 0.5 mL per sec.

- Perfect emulsion gives a look of a homogenous curd. The sound of the homogenizer changes at the point of emulsion breakdown and gives appearance of broken curd.
- Write down the amount of oil required at break point of emulsion.

Calculation

The EC is expressed as the amount of oil emulsified by one g of meat protein.

7. Determination of instrumentation textural value

Tenderness is an important meat quality trait that influences the consumer acceptability. Various factors influencing meat tenderness are type of animal, age, muscle location, connective tissue content, muscle fibre diameter etc. In animal body the tenderest muscle is *Psoas major* and most tough muscle is Sternocephalicus. Tenderness of muscle can be measured both by resistance to mechanical shearing and by palatability test.

7.1 Warner – Bratzler/ Kramer shear force value

7.1.1 Principle

W-B shear force value is an objective measurement of tenderness. It measures the force required to shear the muscle by mechanical means and is calculated by using instrument called Warner-Bratzler Shear Press or Kramer Shear Press.

7.1.2 Apparatus, raw materials and chemicals

- Meat sample, water bath, Warner-Bratzler/Kramer Shear Press apparatus/Texture analyzer, sampling core, LDPE bags.

7.1.3 Procedure

- Cook the meat samples at 80^{0}C for 20 min in a water bath and cool in a refrigerator.
- Prepare samples of 1cm^2 or round samples with a core sampler.
- Place the sample on cutting blade of W-B shear press.
- Switch on the Warner Bratzler/Kramer Shear Press machine.

- Meat sample is cut slowly by the machine blade and the needle is deflected due to force of shearing the sample.
- Take at least ten readings for each sample and calculate the average value.
- Express the shear force value as kg/cm^2.

Note:

1. Sample should be placed perpendicular to the fibre direction for shearing.

7.2 Texture profile analysis (TPA)

Texture as a quality attributes varies among types of food. Consumer products succeed in the marketplace in part because their "textural characteristics" are pleasing to customers. Texture analysis is the mechanical testing of food materials including foods of animal origin and other consumer products in order to measure their physical properties. Now-a-days use of texture analyzers for analysis of food products is most common, though sensory analysis considered more scientific but are subject to wide variability, are labour intensive and therefore expensive. Instrumental methods of assessing texture can be carried out under more strictly defined and controlled conditions. Sensory analysis includes use of the senses of smell, taste, sound and touch. The texture analysers are used to measure many properties, such as hardness, brittleness, spreadability, adhesiveness, tensile strength, extensibility etc, on a vast range of products. The tests also cover those atributes relating to rheology of solid, semi-solid, viscous liquid, powder and granulate materials.

7.2.1 Principle

Different parameters in textural analysis are determined from the force × time or using force × distance plot. Some of the most common parameters analyzed using force × time plot in texture analyzers are Hardness (N) = maximum force required to compress the sample (second peak, F_2); Springiness (cm) = the distance that the product recovered its height during the time that elapsed between the end of the first bite and the start of the second bite; Cohesiveness (A_2/A_1) = the ratio of the positive force area during the second compression (A_2) to the positive area during the first compression (A_1); Gumminess (N) = A_2/A_1×hardness; Chewiness (N cm) = calculated as hardness × cohesiveness× springiness and Resilience = the ratio of area of A_5/A_4.

7.2.2 Apparatus and chemicals

- Texture analyzer equipped with load cell, probe and relevant software.

7.2.3 Procedure

- Place strip of muscles or slices of each sample of 1 × 1 × 1 cm^3 on the compression platform.
- Set the pre-standardized programme in the texture analyzer software attached with the probe and load cell.
- Run the machine with pre-standardized programme [may be set to pre-test speed (2 mm/s), post-test speed (5 mm/s) and test speed (1 mm/s) with a deformation of 3 mm, time (2 s) having a load cell of 500 N].
- Take at least 4-5 sub-samples from each sample subjected to be tested.
- Determine the parameters like hardness (N), springiness (cm), cohesiveness, chewiness and resilience as mentioned earlier or any other parameters from graph developed during analysis.

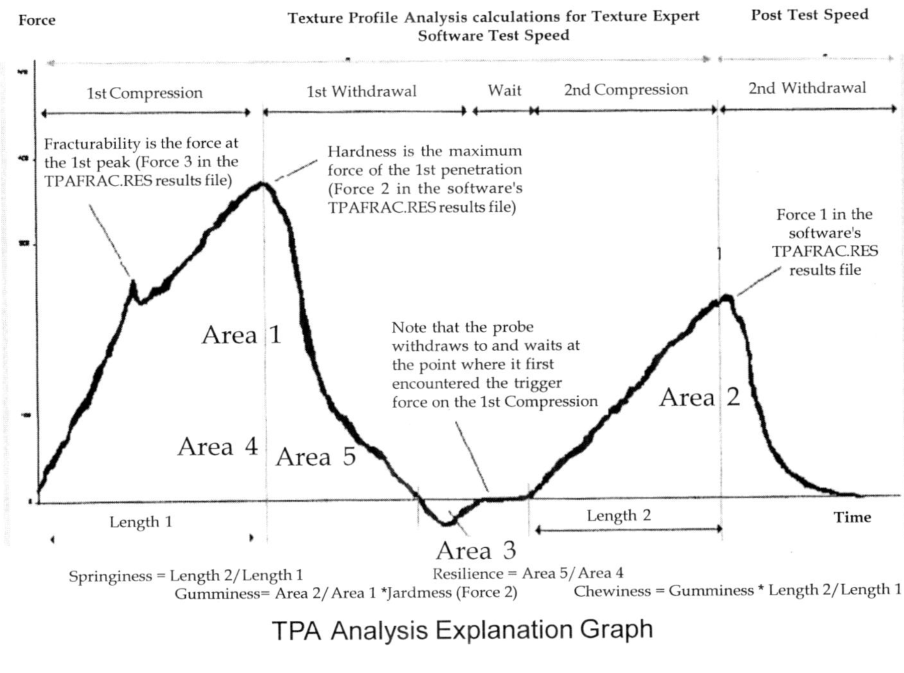

TPA Analysis Explanation Graph

8. Muscle fiber typing (Combined staining for identifying muscle fiber types)

8.1 Principle

Unfixed tissue sections are stained first for metabolic function with NADH and then for physiological function by the acid ATPase reaction.

8.2 Solutions

- Acid Pre-incubation solution: 100 ml $CaCl_2$ (0.18 M), 3 ml Glacial acetic acid, 890 ml H_2O (Adjust pH to 4.3, QS 1 L).

Note:

Even though the pH is adjusted at this step it will need to be adjusted again depending on the species of meat.

- Rinse solution: 12.1g Tris Base, 100 ml $CaCl_2$ (0.18 M), 900 ml H_2O - Adjust pH to 7.8.
- ATPase incubation medium: (Make fresh immediately before use) 40 ml batch 200 ml batch, 2.68 ml 2-Amino 2-Methyl 1-Propanol (1.5 M) 13.40 ml, 4.0 ml $CaCl_2$ 20.00 ml, 0.148 g KCl 0.740 g, 0.0608 g ATP 0.304 g

  32.0 ml H_2O 160.0 ml - Adjust pH to 9.4; incubate tissues to 37^0C.
- NADH incubation solution: (Make fresh daily) 10 ml 0.2 M Tris buffer, pH 7.4, 10 mg Tetranitro Blue Tetrazolium (TNBT), 8 mg Nicotinamide Adenine Dinucleotide, reduced, Filter before use.

Note :

No matter how long you mix this it never seems to go into solution, therefore, it MUST be filtered.

- Tris buffer (pH 7.4): 75 ml .02 M Tris base (12.11 g/500 ml), 126 ml 0.1 M HCl (50 mls of 1 N HCl, QS 500 ml), 174 ml H_2O (As a preservative, add a few drops of Chloroform).
- Ehrlich's hematoxylin stain: 6 g Hematoxylin, 300 ml Ethyl alcohol (absolute), 9 g Aluminum ammonium sulfate, 300 ml H_2O, 300 ml Glycerin (Glycerol), 0.72 g Sodium Iodate, 30 ml Glacial Acetic Acid- Mix and then filter.

Note :

The stain can be reused several times.

- 0.18 M $CaCl_2$: 26.46 g/L,
- 1% (w/v) $CaCl_2$: 10 g/L
- 2% (w/v) $CaCl_2$: 10 g/500 ml
- 2% (v/v) Ammonium Sulfide: 10 ml/500 ml **(Must mix under the hood)**
- 50% (v/v) Ethyl Alcohol.
- Glycerol gelatin (to mount slides): The glycerol needs to be warmed before use. Keep a beaker of water on a hot plate (lowest setting) and keep the glycerol bottle sitting in the beaker while mounting slides.

8.3 Staining sequence

- NADH solution, 45 min. @ 37°C.
- Distilled water, 30 sec.
- Acid pre-incubation solution, 10 min.
- Rinse solution, 2 min.
- ATPase incubation solution, 30 min. @ 37°C.
- 1% $CaCl_2$, 1.5 min.
- 2% $CaCl_2$, 3 min.
- Distilled water, 2 min.
- 2% Ammonium Sulfide, 3 min. (Do this step in the hood)
- Running distilled water, 3 min.
- Hematoxylin, 5 min.
- Running distilled water, 3 min.
- 50% EtOH, 2 min.
- Drain and mount with Glycerol gel.

8.4 Results

Red fibers: Fibers that stain dark purple.

Intermediate fibers: Fibers that stain intermediate.

White fibers: Fibers that stain light purple.

Notes:

- For "cleaner" slides, filter the NADH solution before using it.
- If three fiber types are not identifiable, increase the pH of pre-incubation solution until desired intensity is obtained.

References

Ashmore C.R. and Doerr R. 1971. *Exp. Neurol.* 31: 408.

Davis, G.W., Duston, T. R. Smith, G.C. and Carpenter, Z. C. 1980. *J. Food. Sci.* 45: 880.

Gornall, A.G. Bardanill, C. T. and David, M. M. 1949. *J. Biol. Chem.* 177: 751.

Jermiah, L. E. and Martin, A.H. 1977. *Canadian J Anim Sci.* 57: 7.

Oslon, D.G., Parrish, F.C. Jr. and Stromer, M. H. 1976. *J. Food Sci.*, 41: 1036.

Solomon M.B. and Dunn M.C. 1988. *J. Anim. Sci.* 66: 255-264.

Swift, C.E., Lockett, C and Fryer, A.S. 1961. *Food Technol.* 15: 468.

Tuma *et al.*, 1962. *J. Anim. Sci.* 21(1): 33-36.

□□□

Chapter IV

Assessment of Keeping Quality of Meat

Meat products are highly perishable in nature and need appropriate intervention strategies for their preservation. The preservation technique is most essential for prolonging the shelf life as well as storage of meat and meat products. The processes used in meat preservation are principally concerned with inhibiting microbial spoilage. Preservation minimizes the depreciation of food quality by slowing down or stopping enzymatic, biochemical and physical changes. These may be achieved by controlling temperature, or moisture, and more directly by use of chemicals (bactericidal, bacteriostatics, fungicidal and fungistatics), or even use of physical treatments like irradiation, microwave cooking, high pressure treatment and different packaging techniques. Even then, large portions of meat are wasted due to inadequate handling, processing, distribution and marketing. Many a times these highly priced and nutritious foods undergo decay due to exposure of higher temperature coupled with frequent power cut or inadequate access to refrigerated facilities during transportation and distribution. Since consumers are concern about the quality of meat and meat products received from different points of sale, authentication of these products using reliable tests is required. Keeping quality of the meat can be judged by evaluating, pH, extract release volume (ERV), water activity (a_w), TBARS value, peroxide value, free fatty acid contents, titratable acidity, microbial quality, sensory quality etc. Some of the techniques for evaluation of meat quality are given as under-

1. pH (Trout et al., 1992)

The normal physiological pH of muscular tissue ranges between 7.0-7.2. The ultimate pH of meat is reached to 5.4–5.6 in 18-24 h post-mortem. On storage, there is change in pH of meat and meat products due to metabolites of bacterial action. The deviation in pH is considered as indicator of the quality of meat. pH of meat is measured by different methods, either by digital pH meter or probe pH meter for online carcass pH determination or Nitrazine yellow indicator test or pH paper strip test. The pH of meat sample homogenate is measured either by electronic digital pH meter or by pH paper strips.

1.1 Principle

The pH represents the acidity or alkalinity of a solution or masses. The pH expresses the H^+ or OH^- ion concentration in sample from -2 to 20.

1.2 Apparatus and chemicals

- Tissue homogenizer/Pestle and Mortar, Digital pH meter/pH, Weighing balance, Glass beaker (100 mL).
- Deionized water, paper strips, pH buffer solution (4.01, 7.0 and 9.2).

1.3 Procedure

- Take 10g of minced meat sample free from bone grits, fascia etc in a glass beaker.
- Add 50 ml of de-ionized distilled water to it.
- Homogenize the sample with the help of tissue homogenizer at 7,000 – 10,000 rpm for 1 min. or triturate with pestle and mortar.
- Calibrate the digital pH meter with the different buffer solution.
- Immerse the glass electrode and thermocouple of digital pH meter into meat homogenate.
- Let the reading get stable and note the pH of sample.
- Wipe the electrodes and place into KCl solution as provided with the equipment.
- Alternatively, immerse pH paper strips (pH 5-7) into homogenate and take them out.
- Dry the strips and compare the colour with colour chart.

2. Extract release volume (ERV) (Strange et al., 1977)

2.1 Principle

ERV refers to volume of aqueous extract released by meat / fish homogenate when it is passed through a Whatman filter paper No. 1 for a given period of time. As meat undergoes microbial spoilage, there is a complete hydrolysis of proteins, which significantly decreases the ERV. Therefore, good quality meat has higher ERV value than poor quality meat.

2.2 Apparatus and chemicals

- Tissue homogenizer/Pestle and Mortar, Measuring cylinder, Funnel, Time clock, Glass beaker.
- Whatman Filter paper No. 1, Distilled water.
- Phosphate buffer solution (0.2 M): Mix solutions of 0.2 M Na_2HPO_4 (Mol. wt. 178) and 0.2 M NaH_2PO_4 (Mol wt. 156.1) in ratio of 1:8 and store in refrigerator.
- Working solution of phosphate buffer (0.5 M): Dilute 250 ml of stock solution to 1000 ml with distilled water to get 0.05 M phosphate buffer of 5.8 pH.

2.3 Procedure

- Take 15g of minced meat and blend with 60ml of 0.05 M PBS (pH 5.8) for two minutes in a tissue homogenizer.
- Filter the homogenate through Whatman No1 filter paper.
- Filtration is carried out at 20 ± 4°C for 15 minutes and filtrate is collected in a measuring cylinder.
- Volume of filtrate is taken as a measure of ERV.

Notes:

- Properly homogenize the sample.
- Note the time correctly as results are interpreted on the basis of time
- The good quality meat exudes 25-40 ml of ERV in 15 min. however, poor quality/ spoiled meat exudates less than 25 ml.

3. Water activity (a_w)

3.1 Principle

Water activity (a_w) is the partial vapour pressure of water in a substance divided by vapour pressure of pure water at the same temperature. It is calculated as= p/p_0, Where p is the vapour pressure of water in the substance, and p_0 is the vapour pressure of pure water at the same temperature.

3.2 Apparatus, raw materials and chemicals

- Water activity meter equipped with sensor, sample cup, meat sample

3.3 Procedure

- Fill finely ground meat up to 80 % volume of a moisture free sample cup.
- Place the sample cup into the sample holder.
- Place the a_w sensor on it for five min.
- Beeps of the a_w meter indicate that it is ready with reading.
- At least duplicate reading should be performed for each sample.
- Take the average of reading.

4. Lipid quality

Lipid oxidation is one of the major factors affecting the quality of precooked meat products. Lipid oxidation is influenced by the composition of phospholipids, the amount of polyunsaturated fatty acids, the presence of metal ions, oxygen, haem pigments, mechanical processes, and the addition of salt during processing. Lipid oxidation is initiated when polyunsaturated fatty acids react with molecular oxygen via free radical chain mechanism forming peroxides. Myoglobin oxidation causes discolouration, which influences consumer acceptance in the market place. However, the fatty acid compositions of phospholipid fractions of the muscle cells are especially important in determining the stability of meat, because oxidative changes are initiated from the membrane components of muscle cells. Lipid hydroperoxides formed during the propagation phase of the peroxidation process are unstable and produce various chemicals which adversely affect quality and safety by encouraging coronary heart disease, cancer and stroke. So determination of such compounds in muscle foods is important.

4.1 Thiobarbituric acid reacting substance (TBARS) value

Thiobarbituric Acid (TBA) value/ Thiobarbituric Acid Reactive Substances (TBARS) number is used as an indicator of oxidative rancidity in meat foods. It is highly correlated with oxidized and warmed-over-flavour of meat and meat products. TBA assay measures the amount of malonaldehyde, a secondary metabolite produced mainly from oxidation of polyunsaturated fatty acids in meat sample.

Method-I: Extraction method (Witte et al., 1970)

4.1.1 Principle

TCA solution extracts the malonaldehyde compounds which react with the TBA reagent giving pink colour which is measured spectrophotometrically at 532 nm wavelength and multiplied with value 5.2.

4.1.2 Apparatus, chemicals and reagents

- Spectrophotometer, Blender/homogenizer/pestle and mortar, Hot Water bath, Distilled water, Graduated cylinder/volumetric flask, Test tubes with stand.
- 2-thiobarbituric acid reagent and trichloroacetic acid.

4.1.3 Procedure

- Take 10 g of meat sample and blend it finely with 50 ml of 20% TCA in a warning blender/ homogenizer for 2 minutes. The pestle & mortar can also be used for homogenization of sample.
- Allow 10 min for extraction.
- Filter the extract through Whatman filter paper No 42.
- In a test tube take 3 ml of this extract, mix with equal volume of 0.005 M TBA reagent.
- Prepare blank sample by mixing 20% TCA with equal volume of 0.005 M TBA reagent.

- Keep the mixture at 27°C for 16 h under dark or alternatively boil for 35 minutes in a water bath and cool the test tubes.
- Measure the absorbance at 532 nm by a spectrophotometer.
- TBA value is calculated by comparing the absorbance of test sample with a standard graph prepared by using known concentrations of malonaldehyde.
- Alternatively it can be directly calculated by multiplying O.D. with **K value i.e. 5.2.**

Notes:

1. Properly blend the meat sample with TCA.
2. Run blank along with meat sample with similar treatment.
3. For preparing standard graph, dissolve 0.3055 g of 1, 1, 3, 3 tetra-ethoxy-propane (TE) in 100 ml of 95 % ethanol (Conc. 1mg/mL malonaldehyde).
4. Prepare a standard graph by using different concentration of malonaldehyde.

Method-II: Distillation method (Tarladgis et al., 1960)

4.1.4 Principle

Heating of meat sample in acidic solution vaporize malondehyde compounds whcih circulate through condenser are collected for chemical reaction with TBA reagents.

4.1.5 Apparatus, chemicals and reagents

- Spectrophotometer, Waring Blender/homogenizer, Pestle and mortar, Volumetric flask 100mL, Water bath, Kjeldahl flask 500 mL, Kjeldahl distillation apparatus, Graduated cylinder 100mL, Glass stopper tubes 50 mL capacity, Glass beads, Whatman filter paper No.1, Meat sample, Paraffin wax, 2-thiobarbituric acid reagent (0.1 % solution), 6N Hydrochloric acid.
- 1,1,3,3, tetraethoxypropane 1mg/ml stock solution- prepared by dissolving 0.3055 g of TEP in 100 ml of 95 % alcohol.
- Working standards of 1,1,3,3 tetraethoxypropane (ranging from 0.6µg to 1.8µg/mL) Prepared by taking 0.3 ml of stock solution

of TEP making the volume to 100 mL with distilled water, which contained 3μg/mL.

4.1.6 Procedure

- Weigh 10 g of meat and mix properly with 50 mL chilled distilled water in a waring blender for 2 minutes.
- Transfer the mixture quantitatively into a Kjeldahl flask of 500 mL capacity by washing with additional 45 mL distilled water.
- Add 5 mL of 6N HCl solution to bring the pH to 1.6.
- Add small amount of paraffin wax and few glass beads in the Kjeldahl flask in order to prevent bumping.
- Assemble the apparatus and heat the flask at the lowest heat on the Kjeldahl distillation apparatus.
- Collect 50 mL of distillate and mix thoroughly.
- Filter 5 mL of distillate and transfer it to a 25 mL glass stopper test tube.
- Add 5 mL of TBA reagent, stopper the tubes, mix contents and finally immerse in a boiling water bath for 35 min.
- Prepare a blank with distilled water and heat like the sample.
- Cool the tubes in tap water for 10 min
- Measure the OD of the sample against blank at 538 nm wavelength

Calculations

$$\text{TBA value (mg malonaldehyde/kg)} = OD_{538\text{ nm}} \times 7.8 \text{ (factor)}.$$

Notes:

1. Prepare working standard solution of TEP ranging from 0.6 μg to 1.8 μg as per TBA estimation by extraction method described earlier.
2. Take the readings with the help of "Standard TEP curve" and express as mg of malonaldehyde /kg of meat.

4.2 Free fatty acids (FFAs) (Koniecko, 1979)

4.2.1 Principle

Free fatty acids form during oxidation process of fats/lipids is extracted by chloroform and titrated against alchoholic KOH to get pink colour end point. It is calculated and expressed as 'per cent of oleic acid'.

4.2.2 Apparatus and chemicals

- Weighing balance, Pestle and Mortar, Burette, Conical flask, Measuring cylinder.
- Sodium sulphate anhydrous, Whatman filter paper No 1, Chloroform, Ethanol, Potassium hydroxide, Phenolphthalein indicator.

4.2.3 Procedure

- Weigh 5 g of sample, transfer to a pestle and mortar.
- Blend into fine powder using anhydrous sodium sulphate.
- Mix with 30 mL of chloroform for 2 min.
- Filter the slurry through Whatman filter paper No. 1 into a 100 mL conical flask.
- Add about 2 or 3 drops of 0.2 % phenolphthalein indicator solution to the chloroform extract.
- Titrate against 0.1N alcoholic potassium hydroxide to get the pink colour end point.
- Note the quantity (mL) of potassium hydroxide required for titration.

Calculation

$$\text{Free fatty acid (FFA) (\%)} = \frac{0.1 \times \text{ml } 0.1\text{N alcoholic KOH} \times 0.282}{\text{Sample weight (g)}} \times 100$$

4.3 Peroxide value (PV) (Koniecko, 1979)

4.3.1 Principle

Peroxide forms due to auto-oxidation of fat/lipid is extracted by chloroform and titrated against sodium thiosulphate to get end point (non aqueous layer turn colourless). It is calculated and expressed as 'meq/kg of sample'.

4.3.2 Apparatus and chemicals

- Weighing balance, Pestle and Mortar, Burette, Conical flask, Measuring cylinder.
- Sodium sulphate anhydrous, Whatman filter paper No 1, Chloroform, Ethanol, Potassium hydroxide, Phenolphthalein indicator.

4.3.3 Procedure

- Weigh 5 g of meat sample and the blend with 30 mL of chloroform for 2 min in the presence of anhydrous sodium sulphate.
- Filter the mixture using Whatman filter paper No.1.
- Measure 25 mL aliquot of the filtrate, transfer to 250 mL conical flask and then add 30 mL of glacial acetic acid and 2 mL of saturated potassium iodide solution.
- Allow to stand for 2 min with occasional shaking (swirling).
- Add 100 mL of distilled water and 2 mL of fresh 1 % starch solution.
- Titrate the flask contents immediately against 0.1N sodium thiosulphate till the end point reach to colourless (non-aqueous layer turned to colourless).
- Estimate mL of sodium thiosulphate required, calculate and express as meq/kg of the meat.

Calculation

$$\text{PV (meq/kg sample)} = \frac{0.1 \times \text{ml } 0.1\text{N sodium thiosulphate}}{\text{Wt. of sample (g)}} \times 100$$

4.4 Acid value

4.4.1 Principle

Fatty acids present in substantial quantity in animal fats are oleic, palmitic and stearic. Free fatty acids are the products of enzymatic or microbial hydrolysis of lipids and goes on increasing during storage of meat. Flavour deterioration in meat is significant when the acidity of the extracted fat reaches 2-3 % (as oleic acid). The acid value of a fat is the number of mg of potassium hydroxide (KOH) needed to neutralize the free acid in 1 g of fat.

4.4.2 Reagents

- A mixture of equal volume of alcohol (95%) and ether.
- 1% Phenolphthalein in alcohol.
- 0.1 N KOH.

4.4.3 Procedure

- Weigh about 10 g of the oil or fat, accurately into a 250 ml conical flask.
- Add 50 ml of ethanol and ether mixture (1:1), neutralised after the addition of 1 ml of phenolphthalein solution.
- Titrate with N/10 KOH with constant shaking until a pink colour persists for 15 sec.
- Note titre value in ml (A).

Calculation

Acid value = A x 0.00561 x 1000 / Weight in g of substance

5. Protein quality

Protein is the most important component of the meat. It is essential to maintain required amino acids of human diet. Many a times such component undergoes degradative changes due to oxidation or hydrolysis by bacterial/inherent enzymatic proteolysis. So its determination in muscle food content is important by valid tests.

5.1 Protein oxidation (Jia et al., 2012)

5.1.1 Principle

Oxidation of proteins gives rise to production of sulfhydryl (SH) content which react with the DTNB [5, 5'-dithiobis-(2-nitrobenzoic acid) and produce colour compound that are determined spectrophotometrically.

5.1.2 Apparatus and chemicals

- Pestle and mortar, Centrifuge machine, Centrifuge tube, Whatman filter paper No. 1.
- Disodium phosphate, sodium dihydrogen phosphate, EGT, EDTA, Tris-base, Glycine, 5, 5'-dithiobis-(2-nitrobenzoic acid).

5.1.3 Procedure

- Weigh 0.5 g of product sample, transfer to a pestle and mortar and then triturate with five volumes of (2.5 ml) of phosphate buffer solution (PBS).
- Centrifuge at 2000 rpm for 10 min.
- Filter the supernatant through Whatman filter paper No. 1.
- Take 0.5 mL of filtrate in a separate test tube, mix with 4 mL EGT buffer (pH 8.2) containing 4mM EDTA, 0.1M glycine and 0.09M Tris base.
- Centrifuge at 12,000 rpm for 15 min.
- Take an aliquot of 4.0 ml of the supernatant in a separate test tube and then add 0.5 mL of 10mM DTNB [5, 5'-dithiobis-(2-nitrobenzoic acid)].
- Incubate the mixture at 27±2°C for 30 min under dark.
- Read the absorbance at 412 nm.
- Calculate the -SH concentration in samples using a molar extinction coefficient of 13,600 per M/cm, and express to nmole/g of sample.

5.2 Tyrosine value (Strange et al., 1977)

5.2.1 Principle

Most of the tyrosine in meat is produced due to hydrolysis of meat proteins. Hydrolytic changes in meat during storage can be caused either due to bacterial proteolysis or automatic changes by inherent tissue enzymes. Tyrosine value increases with advanced spoilage but was not very sensitive to changes during early stage of spoilage.

5.2.2 Apparatus and chemicals

- Spectrophotometer, Pestle and mortar, Whatman filter paper No 42.
- Tyrosine standard, Trichloroacetic acid, Folin and Ciocalteus reagent, Sodium hydroxide.

5.2.3 Procedure

- Weigh accurately 20 g minced meat sample, transfer to a pestle and mortar and then blend with 50 mL of precooled 20 % TCA solution for 2 min.
- Transfer the contents quantitatively to a beaker by rinsing with 50 mL cold distilled water, mixed and filtered through a Whatman filter paper No 42.
- Take 2.5 mL of TCA extract and mix with equal amount of distilled water.
- Mix with 10 mL of 0.5 N Sodium hydroxide.
- Add 3 mL of diluted Folin and Ciocalteus reagent (1 volume concentrated F and C reagent + 2 volumes distilled water) and mix again.
- Allow to stand in a dark place at room temperature for 15 min for proper colour development.
- Take optical density at 700 nm.
- Calculate tyrosine value and express as mg tyrosine per g of meat by referring to a standard calibration curve.

5.3 Free amino acid content

5.3.1 Principle

- Free amino acid content is determined in the non-protein nitrogen (NPN) fraction by ninhydrin reagent.

5.3.2 Reagent

- Ninhydrin reagent - dissolve 0.3 g of ninhydrin in 97 ml of N-butanol and 3 ml of glacial acetic acid.

5.3.3 Procedure

- To 10 ml of sarcoplasmic fraction of protein add 5 ml 10% TCA to precipitate the true proteins.
- Centrifuge the contents for 15 minutes and decant the supernatant.
- Dilute 2 ml of supernatant with distilled water adjusting the pH to 7 and making the final volume to 100 ml in a volumetric flask.
- Take 2 ml and add 1 ml ninhydrin reagent and heat in a water bath (70^{0}C) for about 10 minutes.
- Cool and measure the absorbance at 530nm in a spectro-photometer.
- The concentration of free amino acids can be arrived by the regression equation constructed from reference value.

Preparation of regression equition

- Dissolve 65.5 mg of Leucine in 100 ml distilled water.
- Transfer 0.5, 1, 1.5, 2.0 and 2.5 ml into 100 volumetric flask and follow the steps as above.
- Plot a graph for the known concentration of Leucine and construct a regression equation for calculation.

5.4 Total volatile nitrogen (TVN)

5.4.1 Principle

In most species of fish volatile bases consist of ammonia and amines. In meat trimethylamine is present in minute quantities and total volatile nitrogen mainly consists of ammonia. As ammonia production due to de-amination of protein increases during spoilage, its estimation is a simple method to monitor the quality lean meat. Meat extract is treated with relatively weak alkali and the volatile base is distilled over standard acid or boric acid.

5.4.2 Reagent

- Boric acid reagent- dissolve 5 g boric acid in 100 ml of 95% alcohol, add 350 ml of water.

- Add 5 ml of indicator (0.066% methyl red and 0.33 % bromocresol green in alcohol).
- Add 40% NaOH till a faint reddish colour appear.
- Make the volume upto 500 ml with alcohol.

5.4.3 Procedure

- Homogenise 100 g meat with 2.5 -5 g trichloroacetic acid in a porcelain basin to make fine slurry and cover with aluminum foil for 30 min.
- Filter on a Buchner funnel through a Whatman paper No.5.
- Keep the filtrate under refrigeration until use.
- The diffusion is carried out in triplicate with a blank of 2 ml of Boric acid solution.
- Pipette 1 ml of filtrate into the other compartment by sliding the lid.
- Add 1 ml of saturated potassium carbonate solution through the gap and close the lid quickly.
- Rotate the dish on an oscillating table and allow the diffusion of volatile nitrogen at 37°C for 3 hrs, during incubation rotate the dish 2-3 times.
- Titrate boric acid in the central compartment with 0.02 N H_2SO_4 and calculate the total volatile nitrogen.

Mg TVN/100 g meat = Reading of burette x normality of acid used for titration x 14 x 100 = X x 0.02 x 14 x 100.

6. Estimation of acidity

6.1 Total acidity (Lactic acid)

6.1.1 Principle

Total acidity or titrable acidity expressed as lactic or acetic acid may be used as an indirect measure of bacterial growth in brines and liquid foods. Measurement of acid present may be accomplished by titration of a suitable quantity of sample with 0.1 N NaOH to the phenolphthalein end point (pH 8.3). Total acidity is the amount of standardized 0.1N NaOH used to neutralize the acidity of a meat sample to the pH level of phenolphthalein used as indicator.

6.1.2 Apparatus and chemicals

- Weighing balance, Pestle and Mortar, Burette, Conical flask, Measuring cylinder.
- Sodium hydroxide, Whatman filter paper No 2, Phenolphthalein indicator.

6.1.3 Procedure

- Weight 10 g of meat sample and then transfer to a pestle and mortar.
- Homogenize with 200 mL of distilled water, make up volume to 250 mL in volumetric flask and thereafter filter the slurry through Whatman filter paper No. 2.
- Collect 25 mL of filtrate and to it add 75 mL of distilled water.
- Add three drops of phenolphthalein and titrate against 0.1N NaOH.
- Measure the amount of 0.1 N NaOH requires in titration.
- Calculate the total acidity and express as % lactic acid.

Calculations

$$\text{Total acidity (\% lactic acid)} = \frac{\text{mL NaOH} \times \text{N NaOH} \times \text{meq wt. of lactic acid} \times 100)}{\text{Weight of sample in g}}$$

(meq. wt. of lactic acid = 90/1000= 0.09)

6.2 Titrable acidity (TA) (Shelf and Jay, 1970)

In determining the organic acids in foods titrable acidity has been repeated to be of more value than pH alone, as the latter is a measure of hydrogen ion concentration and organic acids do not ionize completely. It has further been reported that in measuring the titrable acidity the amount of acid that is capable of reacting with a known amount of base is determined.

6.2.1 Principle

Total acidity or titratable acidity expressed as lactic or acetic acid may be used as an indirect measure of bacterial growth. Measurements of acid present may be accomplished by titration of a suitable quantity of sample with 0.1 N NaOH to the phenolphthalein end point (pH 8.3).

6.2.2 Apparatus and chemicals

- Waring blender/pestle and mortar, volumetric flask 250 ml, Whatman's filter paper No. 2, Burette 50 ml, conical flask 100 mL.
- 1% Phenolphthalein indicator, 0.1 NaOH.

6.2.3 Procedure

- Weigh 10 g of meat sample and blend with 200 mL of distilled water in Waring blender/pestle and mortar.
- Make up to 250 mL in volumetric flask and mix well.
- Filter the slurry through Whatman filter paper No.2.
- Take 25 mL of filtrate, add 75 ml distilled water and mix well.
- Add three drops of 1% phenolphthalein indicator solution and titrate against 0.1N NaOH.
- Measure the amount of 0.1 N NaOH used in titration, calculate total acidity and express as % lactic acid.

Calculation

$$\text{Total acidity (\% lactic acid)} = \frac{\text{mL of 0.1 N NaOH} \times 0.1 \times \text{meq wt. of lactic acid} \times 100}{\text{Weight of sample in g}}$$

$$\text{meq. wt. of lactic acid} = \frac{90}{1000} = 0.09$$

7. Glycogen content

Glycogen, a polysaccharide is found in the liver, muscle, kidneys and other tissues but is notably absent from brain. It is the chief storage carbohydrate of muscle and the available ready source of substrate for rapid glycolsis in activity. During extremely active muscular work skeletal muscle uses its glycogen as energy source via glycolsis. During recovery some of the lactate formed in the muscles is transported to the liver and rebuilt to form blood glucose, which returns to the muscles to replenish their glycogen store. On hydrolysis with amylase, it yields maltose and with acid it yields glucose. It thus resembles starch and dextrin in these respects but differ significantly in molecular architecture. In the glycogen molecule the component glucose residues are linked in chains by α-1, 4 and 1, 6 glycoside bonds to give a highly branched structure.

Glycogen is soluble in cold water to form an opalescent solution and ordinarily gives a red colour with iodine, although some forms of glycogen which give blue or purple colour with iodine are known. These colour differences are apparently related to the extent of chain branching, the blue colour representing relatively unbranched chains and the red colour to the highly branched chains.

7.1 Principle

Glycogen present in the meat tissue extracted and saturated using Na_2SO_4 but precipitated when mixed with ethanol. It is re-precipitated by 95% ethanol. On acid hydrolysis by HCl or H_2SO_4, reducing sugar D-glucose is liberated which is determined by means of Anthrone Method. Red colour obtained is estimated in a colorimeter at 620 nm to the concentration of D-glucose.

7.2 Apparatus and chemicals

- Pestle and mortar, Water bath, Colorimeter, Heating assembly.
- 30% KOH, Saturated Na_2SO_4, 95% ethanol, 0.6M or 5 M HCl or H_2SO_4, 0.5M NaOH (Phenol red), Glucose standard solution containing 111 μg or 0.5 μM (90μg).
- **Anthrone Reagent**: Dissolve 0.2g of authrone in 100 ml of 95% H_2SO_4. This should be prepared fresh or kept in the refrigerator for not more than 2 days.

7.3 Procedure

- Weight 1 g of meat sample and make powder in a pestle and mortar.

- Take 100 mg of powdered tissue; boil in 3mL of 30% KOH for 20 to 30 min or until the tissue dissolve completely.
- Precipitate the glycogen by adding 0.5 mL of saturated Na_2SO_4 and 3.5 ml of 95% ethanol.
- Heat again until the mixture boils.
- Cool the mixture, centrifuge at 3000 rpm at 4 °C and discard the solution.
- Dissolve the sediment in 2 mL water and re-precipitated with 2-5 ml of 95% ethanol.
- Hydrolyze the collected sediment for 2 to 2.5 h in 6 mL of 0.6 M HCl or H_2SO_4 or for 30 min in 2 mL of 5 M acid in a boiling water bath.
- Cool the hydrolyzate, neutralize with 0.5 M NaOH (Phenol red) and make up volume to 50-100 mL or dependent on the expected glycogen content.
- For the Anthrone method, take 5mL of neutralized hydrolyzate (containing 15 to 150 µg of glucose) into a test tube.
- Take another tube receives 5mL of glucose standard containing 111 µg or 0.5 µM (90 µg), a third one contains 5 mL water to serve as a blank.
- Immerse the tubes in cold water and add 10 mL of anthrone reagent.
- Cover the tubes with glass marbles and heat for 10 min in boiling water, cool immediately and read in a colorimeter at 620 nm.
- Calculate the glycogen content of the tissue keeping in mind that 1 g of glycogen yields 1.11 g of glucose on hydrolysis. The glucose standard can be made up with allowance for this.

Notes:

- Original muscle composition should be preserved as much as possible by rapid cooling using isopentane, cooled in liquid nitrogen or Freon cooled in liquid air.
- The tissue should be powdered at liquid nitrogen temperature using cooled mortar or by high speed shaking for about one min

in a stainless cartridge with a steel ball at liquid nitrogen temperature.

8. Microbial quality

Meat and meat products are prone to be contaminated with one or another type of bacteria during various processing steps. In the process of converting live animals into meat, microbial contamination of carcass surfaces is unavoidable. Generally, total bacterial load is estimated in meat products to know the sanitary condition under which meat is produced, processed and marketed. While most of the microflora transferred to the carcasses during the slaughtering process is non-pathogenic, there is a possibility that pathogens such as Salmonella spp., *Escherichia coli* O157:H7, *Campylobacter* spp. and *L. monocytogenes* may be present and it represents one of the most critical quality and safety issues faced by the meat industry. Moreover, during recent years with the increase in global trade and awareness of the consumers of the hygienic quality of the meat, international attention is being focused on ways to improve the microbial quality and safety of foods. However, to evaluate the effectiveness of any intervention strategies, it is necessary to know the microbial status of the product before and after implementation of the intervention. The microbial contaminants encountered in fresh buffalo meat from domestic slaughter-houses in India were of 4.8–5.49 log cfu/g for standard plate counts (SPC), 1.6–3.7 log cfu/g for psychrotrophic counts (PTC) and 2.66–4.8 log cfu/g for *Enterococcus faecalis* counts (EFC), respectively. The incidences of pathogens like Salmonella spp., VTEC, and *L. monocytogenes* were recorded up to 9%, 27% and 5.5%, respectively (Biswas *et al.*, 2008).

8.1 Properties of good sample

- Ideal sample should be identical in all properties with the bulk of material.
- It should be large enough for all types of subsequent, intended determinations.
- Size of samples varies from material and type of analysis.
- It should be packed and stored in such a way, that no significant change occurs from moment of sampling till analysis.

8.2 Microbiological sampling of meat/ poultry products

8.2.1 Fresh dressed meat/ poultry

Sample may be drawn by any of the following methods:

- Swab method: A sterile cotton swab is immersed in sterile saline or peptone water and applied over the surface of meat on specific portions e.g. $1cm^2$, $2cm^2$, $4cm^2$ etc at different places. After swabbing the surface, dip the swabs back in sterile diluent solution and break the stick at about ½″ above the swab. Shake the tubes vigorously to discharge the organisms.
- Triturate method: Samples are taken from different part of meat by using sterile knife or scissors. Generally, 10 g of meat is cut using sterile knife and meat sample is blended with sterile saline using sterile pestle and mortar.
- Direct rinse method: Place the meat portion/dressed poultry in a sterile polyethylene bag containing sterile diluents (1:10). With the help of a stomacher the meat sample is homogenized to make a meat homogenate. Known volume of this homogenate is used for microbial evaluation.

8.2.2 Meat/ Poultry products

The microbiological procedures can be followed as mentioned earlier but some specific precautions should be taken for different type of meat and meat products.

- Frozen meat: Frozen sample is rejected if it reaches the laboratory in thaw condition because microbial load might have increased during transition. Thaw the frozen sample in a water bath at 45°C for not more than 30 minutes or thaw at room temperature for 2-4 hours. Never refreeze the sample. Drip collected during thawing can also be used for microbial analysis.
- Cooked meat: Remove the sample in cooked meat as in fresh meat. Generally, large area for swab is used due to lower microbial load in cooked meat.
- Deboned meat: Any of the earlier method can be used.
- Canned meat: Examine the cans for abnormalities such as flipper, soft swell, hot swell and leakage etc. Remove these abnormal cans and determine microbial loads and isolate the microbes. Incubate normal cans at 35°C for 10 days and examine daily. In

case cans do not develop any change till 10 days terminate the analysis. Before opening cans heat the area with a burner and open with pasteurized device. Transfer contents immediately to selected media under laminar flow chamber. Do not flame swells as they may burst. Instead use chlorine solution.

8.3 Preparation of homogenate and serial dilution

- Sterilize diluents (normal saline solution or 0.1% peptone water) in autoclave at 121°C, 15 lbs pressure for 15 minutes.
- Take 9 mL of sterile diluent into the pre-sterilized test tubes.
- Take 10 g sample and add 90 mL of sterile diluent, prepare homogenate with help of sterile pestle and mortar to get 10^{-1} dilution.
- Add 1 mL of meat homogenate/stock solution (swab method) into it with sterilized pipette. Shake it gently.
- Take 1 mL of mixture by another pipette and add it to next test tube with 9 mL diluent solution and subsequently make tenfold dilutions (1:10, 1:100, 1:1000 and so on).

8.3.1 Standard plate counts

Standard Plate Count/Total viable count represent the total bacterial load of meat. It estimates the total number of viable bacteria, which grows into colonies under given conditions of media and temperature. The numbers of colonies appear per g of sample may be slightly less than actual number of bacteria present in the sample because some bacteria require special nutrients and temperature for their growth. Standard plate count agar is used for determination of SPC. For this, weigh 23.5 g of plate count agar (standard methods agar Hi-Media), suspend in 1000 ml of glass distilled water followed by boiling to dissolve the medium completely and sterilized by autoclaving at 15 lbs pressure (121°C) for 15 min. Final pH of the medium was 7.0± 0.2 at 25°C.

8.3.1.1 Procedure

- Inoculate 1 mL from a dilution in pre-marked sterile Petri dish in duplicate.
- Add 15-20 mL of sterile molten media (PCA or TGYA) at 44-48°C in aseptic condition.

- Mix it gently for uniform distribution of sample by rotating the Petri plates in circular and side way rotation.
- Allow to stand until the media solidify.
- After solidification, invert the Petri plates.
- Incubate the plates at 35°C for 48 hours in an incubator.
- Count the number of colonies with the help of colony counter and represent the results in colony forming units/g of sample by multiplying number of colonies with dilution factor.

8.3.2 Psychrotropic plate count

- Prepare the plates in similar manner as described for standard plate count but they should be incubated at 4±1°C for 7 days.
- Count the colonies and express as $\log_{10}$ cfu /g of sample.

8.3.3 Escherichia coli count

- Mac Conkey Agar (MCA) is used to determine *Escherichia coli* in meat sample as recommended by Bureau of Indian Standard (BIS) for isolation and differentiation of lactose fermenting enteric bacteria (*E. coli*).
- For media preparation (Hi-Media) weigh 55.07 g of MCA, suspend in 1000 mL of glass distilled water followed by boiling to dissolve the medium completely and then sterilized by autoclaving at 15 lbs pressure (121°C) for 15 min and cooled to 50°C.
- Final pH of the medium should keep 7.5 ± 0.2 at 25°C.
- Use pour plate method for inoculation of suitable sample dilution and incubate the plates at 35±2°C for 48 h.
- Count pinkish sharp colonies with about 0.5 mm diameter for presumptive determination of *Escherichia coli* and express as $\log_{10}$ cfu/g of the sample.

8.3.4 Staphylococcus spp. count

- For media preparation take 63.0 g of Baird Parker Agar base (Hi-Media), suspend in 950 mL of glass distilled water followed by boiling to dissolve the medium completely and sterilized by autoclaving at 15 lbs pressure (121°C) for 15 min and cooled to 50°C.

- Add aseptically 50 mL of concentrated egg yolk tellurite emulsion and one vial of Baird Parker (BP) sulpha supplement and mix well before pouring.
- Final pH of the medium should be around 7.0± 0.2 at 25°C.
- Follow pour plate method for inoculation of suitable sample dilution, incubate the plates at 35±2°C for 48 h, and finally count viable colonies (Dark centered colonies surrounded by white rings) and express in $\log_{10}$ cfu/g of sample.

8.3.5 Total coliforms count

- Violet Red Bile Glucose Agar (VRBGA) is used for determination of total coliforms.
- The procedure of plating is similar as stated as above.
- Count red to pink colonies of 0.5 mm in diameter and express as $\log_{10}$ cfu/g of sample.

8.3.6 Salmonella spp. count

- For determination of *Salmonella* spp. count, Brilliant Green Agar is used.
- The procedure of plating is similar stated as above.
- Count the light pink colonies of 0.5 mm in diameter and express as $\log_{10}$ cfu/g of sample.

8.3.7 Yeast and mould count

- Surface plate method is most suitable for determination of yeast and mold count.
- For this spread over 0.1mL volume of inoculums of suitable dilutions on the surface of the pre-poured Petridish with potato dextrose agar (PDA) media.
- Maintain pH of the media to 3.5 using sterile 10% tartaric acid.
- Incubate the plates at 25°C for 5 days, and finally count the colonies and express as $\log_{10}$ cfu/g of sample.

Notes:

1. Always mark the Petri plates on the base, never on the lid.
2. The temperature of molten agar while pouring should not exceed 45°C.
3. The care should be taken while mixing the media and sample that it should not spill over the plates.
4. Sterilize the laminar flow chamber properly before proceeding with the experiment.
5. Always count the plates with colonies between 30-300.

9. Sensory evaluation (Keeton, 1983)

Sensory evaluation is the scientific way of evaluation of meat products through use of human senses such as smell, taste, touch, temperature etc. Human senses act as biological detector, which can perceive taste, smell etc where no signal appears by instrument. Eeven though highly sophisticated instruments are vailable, the importance of sensory evaluation is increasing day by day. Moreover, the instruments analyze only single components, while our senses give us total impression of aroma, taste, temperature and other sensory attributes. In meat science sensory analysis reported to have many applications such as quality control of fresh meat and raw materials, meat products, storage stability test, development of new variety of products, comparison among the different products etc. The sensory evaluation of food products began in the year 1940 by the Scandinavians.

9.1 Difference between sensory and organoleptic evaluation

	Sensory evaluation	Organoleptic evaluation
1.	Sensory testing is scientific way of evaluation of meat products and always meets requirement for the purpose of testing.	Organoleptic testing rarely complies with principles of science with objectivity and reproducibility.
2.	Sensory panel members are selected based on threshold and recognition tests and all they possesses sensitivity and	Organoleptic quality graders usually avoid having their sensory ability checked, although this is basic

	reliable, precise and reproducible rating of smell, often minute differences in sensory perception.	requirement for all testing procedures.
3.	Panel members participate in appropriate training courses and periodic selection tests, working in a panel where test results are analyzed statistically.	Systemic training of organoleptic tester sensory organs is lacking
4.	The characteristics of sensory tester include- measuring with his senses using exact methods such as difference tests, descriptive tests etc.	Organoletic testers feel rather than analyze their impression, relying on experience, confusing quality test with hedonic evaluations, and they allow their evaluations to be influenced by others.

9.2 Requirements of testing conditions for sensory evaluation

It is considered that a single expert is not adequate for quality evaluation of finished products. So, group of trained peoples also called as a panel of member is always selected for quality evaluation of meat products following different sensory attributes. The panel members are directed by a panel leader having good sensory abilities. It is recommended that all interested persons of both sexes regardless of their age can participate in test panel. However, persons with abnormal olfactory and gustatory sensitivity, perfumery to which men and women react differently, and highly enthusiastic persons could be restricted from product testing. Younger persons may have more taste buds, whereas, older persons can concentrate better thereby balancing the results.

Smokers and non-smokers are both suitable as there are sensitive and less sensitive persons in both groups. When smokers stop smoking they become more sensitive to the odour and taste of spoiled food products. At the beginning of a training course it is not recommended that smokers be asked to stop smoking or they may lost interest in sensory analysis. But they should not have cigarette, cigar or pipe in their mouth at the moment of product testing. Further, eating of highly spiced foods, taking drink with lingering aftertaste and sucking candies or chewing gum have to be avoided before test. A test should not be started for 30 min after such activities. Persons suffering from shore throat, cold etc should not participate in a test. Untrained housewives and office personnel are not suited for laboratory work. The success of sensory tests depends upon the exact sample preparation. Therefore, basic laboratory training is absolutely necessary for personnel.

The use of strong smelling cosmetics has to be avoided and attention paid to bodily hygiene. Hands should be washed with odorless soaps. Persons working in a laboratory with strong smelling substances should not participate as laboratory odours absorbed by their clothing can disturb other persons and influence their own results. The test subjects should not come to the test in a hurry. As sensory evaluation encourages intense concentration by panel members, disturbances such as noise, off-odours etc must be avoided. Test subjects should not have chance to influence each other by facial expressions or orally conveyed results. Test must be written down on test sheets and presented to the panel leader. However, the number of test subjects depends upon the problem to be solved and the respective test method. The flavor profile method use about five panel members, while for other analytical tests, such as difference tests, at least ten persons should be available. For statistical analysis it is advantageous to have 20-30 test subjects. Hedonic scale with untrained consumers 30 to 50 persons should participate.

9.3 Sensory panel room

1. Panel area should be separated from sample preparation area, free from external & cooking odors.
2. Sample transfer mechanism avoiding odour transfer.
3. Odors from other panelists to be minimized e.g. cosmetics, tobacco etc., on that day avoid (hand cream, hair/body spray, lotion etc).
4. Sinks, drain pipe, water odour avoid, (deionised or double distilled).
5. Materials non porous, no odors, neutral colour (off white) no pattern not collect dirt or mold.
6. Room temperature 22-24^{0}C, RH-45-55%.
7. Minimize noise level- external (traffic) or internal.

8. No communication (visual or oral) between panelists. If one panelist comments like or dislike others may be influenced.
9. Consistent & appropriate light 70-80 ft/candle, shadow less for meat foods–red filtered light-to avoid visible effect of cooking method.
10. Minimize physical discomfort-seating, space etc.
11. Unbiased presentation of samples.
12. Preparation of samples affect sensory attributes e.g. cooking method, serving temperature, holding time, interval from cooking to serving, etc.

9.4 Time of taste: Depends upon the sample

1. Taste subjects are more sensitive when they are hungry.
2. Lunch time should be avoided for taste panel.
3. For meat, fish etc., ideal time is late morning, afternoon, at least 1.5hr after lunch.
4. Tea /Coffee may be given after breakfast or 1/2hr after lunch.

9.5 Development of Panel

9.5.1 Selection of Panel Members

Selection of panelists is critical to obtain reliable sensory data. Select panelist from internal sources of company/institute than external panelists.

Advantage

- No monetary reward required
- Reduces cost of sensory analysis
- Panelists are already on location – no travel
- More diverse demographics than external.

Disadvantage

- Panelists contributing to manufacture of product may be biased, they may be
- Familiar with product being evaluated
- Working duty may interfere with sensory panel duty.

9.5.2 Pre-screening interview

- Describe the job in detail – tasting of meat, scale, scoring.
- Ascertain availability – daily, weekly, monthly etc.
- Determine the interest – liking meat, variety, eating out.
- General state of health – food allergies, cold or sinus, dental or gum disease, mouth sore, diabetic, kidney or coronary disease, any condition affecting any senses.
- Explain the importance of sensory program.
- Interview determines reliability, interest, availability, and health– accepted or rejected. Do not accept if not fully fit as per requirements. If accept it may affect efficiency – e.g., a person with mild interest – frequently absent.

9.5.3 Screening tests

It is to determine sensory acuity and ability to follow directions. It is done in four phases.

- Example for screening tests is given as under-
  - *Scaling & Judgement*:

    Mark on the line the proportion of area shaded in the figure. None-All
  - *Sensory acuity/discrimination*

    a) Cotton balls dipped in different oils with different aroma kept in glass jars.

    b) Triangle tests with sample having differences in juiciness, tenderness or flavour.
  - *Ranking or rating:*

    Making solution of sugar at ascending order of concentration ask to rank them by sipping from cup.
  - *Personal Interview:*

    Interest – very high

    Expectations – time, pay, social contact, commitment

Decisions after screening test:

- Accept for the next phase of testing
- Reject the person
- Continue testing

A person should be accepted in all the four phases before accepted for training. If a person is late for screening, reject; he will be late during testing also. Do not accept inferior people, better to have fewer reliable, repeatable panelists than having more numbers unreliable & less efficient.

9.5.4 Training of sensory panelists

The goal to familiarize with test procedures.

- To improve ability to recognize/identify sensory attributes.
- To improve sensitivity and memory for sensory attributes ultimately to have precise and consistent judgments.

Number of Panelists- depends on (a) familiarity with the product and procedures, (b) expected differences between products, (c) 20% extra, for drop out due to many reasons.

- First Session: Educate about general biology of muscle foods viz. muscle fibre structure, connective tissue, fat coating etc.
  - How the Olfactory senses work?
  - Four basic tastes, their location in tongue.
  - Sensory attributes of meat & meat products.
- Main Sessions: To familiarize panelists with test procedures. Techniques to be presented are :
  - How to chew a sample?
  - How to expectorate the sample –vs – swallowing?
  - How to rinse mouth between each sample?
  - Methods of evaluation – viz. -scale to be used, - anchor points for the scale, - score sheet, terminology to be used.

The type of training needed for panelist depends on the objectives of the study. Muscle foods are evaluated mainly by two types of sensory panels. That is difference testing or descriptive testing. Selection of panelists and amount of training required varies with the type of sensory task.

- Generally they are required to pass through the threshold test for 4 basic tastes.
- Through training and experience they understand judging techniques and critical analysis.
- For meat products panelist should develop the ability to judge one attribute at a time without the influence of other attributes.

Guidelines

1. Present reference sample for each attribute.
2. Concentrate on one attribute in a session till they are familiar with it.
3. Anchor points on the scale for each attribute and how to scale within attribute.
4. Panelists should score individually, then discuss in a group.
5. Panel leader gives overall score.
6. Panelists should re-evaluate to familiarize.
7. Continue & repeat till consistent results are obtained among panelists, by each panelists.
8. Length of training depends on type of panel, number of attributes, previous experience.

9.5.5 Evaluation and monitoring

- It is ongoing and continuous process, to identify problems of individual panelist, to identify areas for further training for all.

9.5.6 Motivating panelists

- It is important to maintain the interest and motivation of panelist.
    1. Feedback about their performance day to day during training will motivate panelists.
    2. If panel leader discusses the result individually or as group is better.

3. If time is a constraint, data can be posted on a chart (-may lead to misinterpretation).
4. A small treat at the end of each session as a reward (Chocolate, nut, juice, fruit).
5. In case of long series of panel – larger reward – a small party (dinner), gift etc., to appreciate panelists.

9.6 Preparation and presentation of samples

1. Cooking method, serving temperature, humidity etc.
2. Degree of doneness, time length and interval from cooking holding period & temperature.
3. Containers used for storing and preparing.
4. Size or quantity of sample.

   - for whole muscle product (steaks, chops, roasts) 1.27cm^3,
   - ground meat product 1.27 or 2.54 cm^2
   - for texture evaluation of brank furthers – a whole piece,
   - for flavour evaluation of sausages a 2.54 cm section.
5. Temperature of sample can affect sensory perception (because aromatic compounds volatiled more at higher temperature).
6. Samples should have 3 digit random code (to avoid subconscious selection).
7. Use glass or white glazed china for presentation, (to eliminate aromatics or visual attribute on sample).
8. Plastics should be opaque, free from odours and neutral in colour.
9. Samples served in random order to avoid order effect (1st sample ranked high or low).

9.7 Sensory evaluation methods

9.7.1 Objective methods

- They involve use of instruments such as Instron/Texturometer, Warner Bratzler shear Press, Flavour Analyzers, Hunter colour Lab/Colorimeter etc for above-mentioned sensory characteristics.

9.7.2 Subjective methods

- These methods include perception through human senses. It involves the specialized panel or consumer panel for testing the sensory attributes of meat and meat products.
- **Recognition and Threshold tests**: This test is used for training of the panel members for making them familiar to four basic tastes. The serial dilutions in ascending order of 0.01% of all the four tastes (cane sugar-sweet; sodium chloride-salty; tartaric acid/citric acid-sourness; caffeine-bitterness) are prepared.
- **Ranking test:** The objective is to select one or two best samples out of all tested samples. A series of test samples are provided in an ascending or descending order of intensity of specific characteristics. The trainee receives a random order of sample and is asked to rank the samples in order of increasing intensity.
- **Hedonic scaling:** In hedonic scaling, effective responses of like and dislikes are measured on a rating scale. Most popular are 8-point or 9-point Hedonic scale, where 8 or 9 = like extremely and 1 = dislike extremely.

In other way sensory evaluation can be two types (i) Product oriented and (ii) Consumer oriented.

- **Consumer-oriented testing**: It is for knowing likes or dislikes, preferences and acceptability using untrained panels. True consumer panel is selected from a large random population. For this 100-500 people are called in a central place and 50 may be selected on interviews. It is costly and time consuming. Hence, an in-house consumer panels are commonly used before true consumer panel. e. g. Organoleptic test, consumer test. The in-house panels consists of 30-50 untrained people from the organization, who use the product and similar to the target consumer. These results are not good for predicting product performance.
- **Product-oriented testing:** Uses small trained panels to identify difference among similar products. To measure intensity of flavour, texture etc. Usually 5-15 people selected on sensory acuity and trained specially for the task. They should not be used for acceptability test. They are sensitive to small differences; they should keep aside their personal likes & dislikes. e.g., Descriptive testing, difference testing

9.8 Difference test / Descriptive test

- **Paired difference test:** In this test, two samples are provided and the analysis is done for a single attribute. The trainee has to identify the sample having more intensity of the specified attribute.
- **Duo-trio test**: In this test, three samples are presented to trainee. One of them is reference sample and other two are coded samples. The trainee has to identify that among the coded samples, which one is similar or different to reference sample.
- **Triangle test:** In this test, three coded samples are provided to trainee and he has to identify which two samples are same or different from the other sample.

9.8.1 Interpretation

- Threshold value for an average good taste is 0.68% cane sugar solution for sweetness, 0.019% tartaric acid solution for sourness, 0.18% sodium chloride for saltiness and 0.009% caffeine solution for bitterness.

Notes:

- Rinse your mouth with potable water between successive samples.
- Never taste more than six samples continuously to avoid fatigue of taste.
- The ideal time for conduct sensory evaluation of meat and meat product is late morning or late afternoon.
- Never compel any one for sensory evaluation.
- Never perform the sensory evaluation full stomach.

References

Biswas, A. K., Kondaiah, N., Anjaneyulu, A. S. R., Bheilegaonkar, K. N., Mendiratta, S. K., Jana, C., Singh, H. and Kumar, R. R. 2008. *Meat Science* 80: 418–422.

British pharmacopoeia Appendix X-A, p. 1055 (1963).

Jia N., Kong B. H., Liu Q., Diao X. P., Xia X. F. 2012. *Meat Sci.* 91:533–539.

Koniecko, E.S. 1979. *Handbook of Meat Chemistry*. Avery Publishing Group, Inc., Wayne.

New Jersey. pp. 53-55.

Pearson D (1968) *J. Sci . Food Agric.* 19 pp 637.

Rosen, H 1957 Arch.Biochem-Biophysics, 67: 10-15.

Shelf, L.A. and Jay, J.M. 1970. *Appl. Microbiol.* 19(6): 902-905.

Tarladgis, B.G., Watts, B.M., Younathan, M.T. and Dugan, L.R. 1960. *J. AOAC* 37: 44-48.

Trout, E.S., Hunt, M.C., Johson, D.E., Clans, J.R., Castner, C.L. and Kroff, D.H. 1992. *J. Food Sci.* 57: 19–24.

Witte, V.C., Krause, G.F. and Bailey, M.E. 1970. *J. Food Sci.* 35:582-585.

□□□

Chapter V

Methods for Exploration of Meat Colour

Most consumers buy exactly what they want to eat, instead of only what is readily available or affordable. Consumers also frequently look for quality seals and trust marks on meat products, and expect manufacturers and retailers to provide products of high quality. Meat quality, and in particular, lean colour is a complex trait influenced by genetic components, the handling of animals during production, transportation, and slaughtering, and the treatment during processing. Meat purchasing decisions are influenced by color more than any other quality factor. Consumers use discoloration as an indicator of freshness and wholesomeness of meat. Red meat tends to turn brown with time when exposed to air. Meat also tends to spoil with time due to microbial activity, so the browning of meat with time is a rough indicator of spoilage. But these two event browning and spoilage- are largely independent. In modern meat processing practice, meat exposed to air will become brown long before spoilage develops, however, as the connection between browning and spoilage persists, so meat colour remains of prime importance to meat industries throughout the world. The pigment responsible for most of this colour is the protein myoglobin. Meat myoglobin (Mb), is a complex sarcoplasmic haem protein, and comprised of 153 amino acids, and the primary structure of Mb depends upon species. Despite differences in the amino acid sequences, many structural and functional properties of Mb are conserved across livestock species. The primary structure of protein dictates the tertiary structure, which in turn influences interactions with ligands and biomolecules. It is known that Mb primary structure influences meat color stability via mechanisms such as autoxidation, haem retention, structural stability, thermostability, and oxygen affinity. The myoglobin molecule consists of a haematin nucleus attached to protein components of the globulin type: the molecular weight is about 17000. The haematin portion comprises a ring of four pyrrol nuclei co-ordinated with a central iron atom. The iron may exist in both reduced and oxidized forms. In the ferrous form it can combine with oxygen and nitric oxide. The ability to combine with oxygen is lost when the globin portion of the molecule is denatured and the tendency for the iron to oxidize to the ferric form is then greatly increased, but union the iron with nitric oxide is strengthened. The interactions of pH, temperature and post-mortem time also affect the biochemical dynamics of early Mb discolouration and hence darker meat colour. Furthermore, variations in amino acid sequence of Mb influence meat color stability through species specific interactions with small biomolecules like lactate and aldehydes. For Mb, a heme protein with different redox states, this is extremely critical, because Mb stability and aforementioned molecular interactions govern meat color/color stability. So, in this perspective, we need sound analytical tools to better understand meat colour attributes in the delivery of consistent quality meat. The colour of the meat is measure either by visually or more precisely with the help of instruments like colorimeter, spectrophotometer and Lovibond tintometer.

1. Use of Lovibond tintometer (Little, 1975; Froahlich *et al.*, 1983)

1.1 Principle

Lovibond tintometer is used for determination of visual colour score of different food products based on Red, Yellow, Blue and Neutral colour. Each format of the Model F has a complete set of 11 racks containing permanent colour red glass filters. Lovibond® colour scale (Red 0.1-0.9, 1.0 -9.0, 10.0-70; Yellow 0.1-0.9, 1.0-9.0, 10.0-70; Blue 0.1-0.9, 1.0-9.0, 10.0-40; Neutral 0.1-0.9, 1.0-3.0). A sample chamber lined with a white PVC reference, a spare white reference, a pair of spare bulbs and rectangular fused glass cells. Samples from three different places of meat mass were taken in the sample holder and secured against the viewing aperture. The sample colour was matched by adjusting red (a) and yellow (b) units, while keeping the blue units fixed at 1.0. The corresponding colour units are recorded.

1.2 Apparatus and materials

- Lovibond tintometer, sample holder, scissors, cutting board.

1.3 Procedure

- Fill the sample in the rectangular glass cell.
- Switch ON the main and switch ON the button with the equipment.
- Place the sample in sample chamber.
- Adjust the colour using the different scale viewing through the tube, so that the product in the sample field and a white reflective surface in the comparison field are observed side by side, suitably illuminated.
- Take the measurement of different colour scores and record it.
- Switch OFF the button with the equipment.
- Take out the glass cell, clean it and keep it in appropriate place.

Measurements

- Since *a*-value indicates redness and *b*-value for yellowness that are noted and the hue and chroma values determined by using the formula, $(\tan^{-1})$ b/a and $(a^2 + b^2)^{1/2}$, respectively where, a = red unit, b = yellow unit.

Notes:

1. The Lovibond® Tintometer is a precision optical instrument which should be kept clean to preserve its accuracy, even in the harsh operating conditions often encountered.
2. This is why the Model F has been designed to allow easy cleaning and maintenance with the minimum of cost and effort.
3. The instrument includes a white plastic liner in the sample chamber, which should be removed and cleaned occasionally if a spillage takes place.
4. Plastic linear chamber should be replaced at intervals to maintain the whiteness of the interior, an essential feature for accurate colour matching.
5. Separate filters in the racks also simplify cleaning and allow replacement of single glasses (as opposed to complete racks) if required.

2. Spectrophotometric method

2.1 Estimation of total meat pigments (Myoglobin)

2.1.1 Principle

The myoglobin (Mb) is converted to cyanometmyoglobin in the presence of $K_3Fe(CN)_6$ and KCN, oxidizing agents, forming a stable compound. Cyano MetMb gives rise to orange/red colour, which has maximum absorbance at 540 nm.

2.1.2 Materials and reagents

- Minced meat, Pestle and mortar, refrigerator, refrigerated centrifuge, measuring cylinder and spectrophotometer, chilled distilled water, potassium ferricyanide solution (50 mg/ml) and potassium cyanide solution (10mg/ml).

2.1.3 Procedure

- Take 10 g of minced meat sample in a mortar and add 30 mL of chilled distilled water.
- Then homogenize the sample by pestle and mortar and the slurry hold overnight at 4°C.
- Centrifuge the slurry at 5000 rpm for 10 min using refrigerated centrifuge, collect supernatant in 50 ml measuring cylinder and re-extract the residue with 20 ml chilled distilled water.
- Pool the supernatant and add distilled water to make volume up to 50 ml.
- Take 20 ml aliquot and add 0.1 ml $K_3Fe(CN)_6$ (50 mg/ml) and 0.1 ml KCN (10 mg/ml) in to it. Read the OD at 540 nm.

Calculation

$$\text{Total meat pigment (mg/g)} = \text{Optical density} \times \frac{K}{\text{Sample Wt. (g)}}$$

$$K \text{ (Proportionality constant)} = 17000 \times \frac{\text{Vol. in lit}}{E}$$

E (milli molar extinction coefficient of Cyanomyoglobin) = 11.3

11300 = Molar extension coefficient of CyanoMetMb

17000 = equivalent weight of meat pigment (myoglobin)

0.05 = Aliquot in litre

1000 = To convert g to mg

Total pigment (mg/g) = OD × 7.52

2.2 Metmyoglobin content (Krzywicki, 1979)

2.2.1 Principle

Metmyoglobin content of the given meat sample was estimated based on the principle of absorption maxima of myoglobin, oxymyoglobin and metmyoglobin at 525 nm, 572 nm and 700 nm wavelengths.

2.2.2 Materials and chemicals

- Phosphate buffer containing Sodium dihydrogen orthophosphate (NaH_2PO_4: $2H_2O$) and Disodium hydrogen orthophosphate or Sodium pyrophosphate dibasic: dihydrate (Na_2HPO_4: $2H_2O$) and Whatman filter paper No.42
- Spectrophotometer, Refrigerator, Meat homogenizer, Refrigerated centrifuge

2.2.3 Procedure

- Take 3.0 g of minced meat sample and thoroughly mixed with 30 mL 0.04 M cold phosphate buffer (pH 6.8) (sample: buffer, 1:10) for 20 sec.
- Hold the sample homogenate at 4 °C for 1 h and then centrifuge at 10,000 rpm for 5 min.
- Filter the supernatant using Whatman filter paper No.42 and read the optical density (O.D.) at 525 nm, 572 nm and 700 nm.
- Calculate percent metmyoglobin according to the formula of Krzywicki (1979).

Calculation

$$\text{Met Mb (\%)} = [1.395 - \frac{(\text{OD } 572 - \text{OD } 700)}{(\text{OD } 525 - \text{OD}700)} \times 100$$

2.3 Nitroso pigment (Cured meat products)

2.3.1 Principle

The method is based on the extraction of nitroso-pigments from cured products with and acetone-water solvent. With the inclusion of HCl in the solvent, the method can be adopted to measure the total pigments present.

2.3.2 Apparatus and chemicals

- Acetone, Hydrochloric acid, Spectrophotometer, Polypropylene centrifuge tubes, Glass stirring rod, Two Pyrex test tubes, Glass funnels, Watch glasses, Balance

2.3.3 Test for cure pigment

- Take 10 g of finely diced meat sample into a beaker and add 40 mL acetone and 3 mL of distilled water.
- Mix the sample vigorously under the dark for 5 min and the filter through Whatman filter paper No 1.
- Read the OD of the filtrate at 540 nm and then multiply with 290 to obtain nitrosohaematin pigment (ppm) against blank containing 80 % acetone in water.
- For total pigment, take 10 g of meat sample in a polypropylene centrifuge tube.
- Add 40 mL acetone, 2 mL water and 1 mL concentrated HCl.
- Mix the meat thoroughly with the glass-stirring rod.
- Cover the tubes with watch glass and then allow to stand for 1 h under dark.
- Filter through No. 42 Whatman filter paper into a test tube.
- Transfer the filtrate into a corvette, read the optical density at 640 nm and calculate as total pigment.
- A blank should maintain contain 80 parts acetone + 2 parts HCl + 18 parts water.
- Express total haem pigments in ppm by multiplying the OD by 680.

Calculation

$$\text{Conversion (\%)} = \frac{\text{ppm nitroso pigment}}{\text{ppm total pigment}} \times 100$$

Where,

Nitroso pigment (ppm) = O.D. (540 nm) × 290

Total pigment (ppm) = O.D. (640 nm) × 680

Notes:

1. The procedure has been scaled down to a small sample size, therefore, the meat sample should be as homogenous as possible.
2. Filtrate must be crystal clear.
3. Percent conversion is calculated on a theoretically possible 100 percent of all hematin can actually be converted to nitroso-pigment.

References

Froehlich, D.A., Gullet, E.A. and Usborne, W.R. 1983. *J. Food Sci.* 48: 152-154.

Krzywicki, K. (1979). *Meat Sci.* 3:1-10.

Little, A. C. 1975. *J. Food Sci.* 40: 410-411.

❏❏❏

Chapter VI

Methods for Determination of Functional Compounds in Meat Products

1. Antioxidant activity

Antioxidants are organic molecules of either synthetic or natural origin, which can avoid or delay the progress of oxidative rancidity. It is mainly imparted to their phenol-derived structure. Antioxidants work by donating hydrogen to the lipid free radical to reform the fat molecule or by donating one hydrogen to a peroxide free radical to form a hydroperoxide and a stable antioxidant free radical. They "sacrifice themselves" by giving up a hydrogen atom, then rearrange to a stable conformation.

$$A{:}\ H + RO\bullet \rightarrow A\bullet + ROH$$

Antioxidants can be classified according to their protective properties at different stages of the oxidation process since they act by different mechanisms. Natural antioxidants are presumed to be safe and are available in variable amounts in plants such as fruits, leaves, flowers, roots, grains and seeds. Plant phenolics, "phytochemicals" are multifunctional and can act as reducing agents, free radical terminators, metal chelators and singlet oxygen quenchers. Flavonoids and other classes of phenolic compounds are important phytochemicals. Extracts from plants which contribute health benefits to consumers, arising from protection from free radical-mediated deteriorations, and which cause retardation of lipid oxidation have stronger antioxidant activity than that of synthetic antioxidants.

In the recent years, many functional food products are developed which are generally produced either incorporating or supplementing functional ingredients during formulation or processing. Since all the functional foods are rich in many biologically active compounds, their determination through better analytical methods are required to safeguard the term functional. Some of the analytical techniques are given to better understand the antioxidant activity of different meat products as under.

1.1 DPPH (1,1-diphenyl-2-picrylhydrazyl) radical scavenging activity

1.1.1 Principle

The ability to scavenge 1, 1 diphenyl-2picrylhydrazyl (DPPH) radical by added antioxidants is determined. DPPH can make stable free radicals in aqueous or ethanol solution, however, fresh DPPH solution must be prepared before every measurement (Kato *et al.*, 1988).

1.1.2 Apparatus and chemicals

- 250 μM DPPH reagent
- 0.1M Tris-HCl buffer (pH 7.4)
- Ethanol
- Gallic acid standard
- Whatman filter paper No 42
- Spectrophotometer

1.1.3 Procedure

- Weigh 5g of meat products and triturate with 20 ml of ethanol for 2 min.
- Transfer the content quantitatively into a beaker and filter through Whatman filter paper No 42.
- Take 1 ml of the filtrate in a test tube, mix with 1ml of 0.1M Tris-HCl buffer (pH 7.4) and finally add 1 ml of DPPH reagent (250 μM).
- Mix the content gently and then incubate in dark for 20 min.
- Measure the absorbency in time t=0 min (t_0) at 517 nm using a UV-VIS Spectrophotometer.

- Incubate the sample tubes at ambient temperature under dark and then measure the absorbency in time t=20 min (t_{20}).
- Use ethanol as blank sample.

Calculation

- The free radical scavenging activity was calculated as a decreased of absorbency from the equation

Scavenging activity (% inhibition) = $100 - (At_{20}/At_{0}) \times 100$.

- Calculate the gallic acid equivalent (200 - 600 μM/ml) for comparing scavenging activity with standard antioxidant after calibration of standard curve as given under.

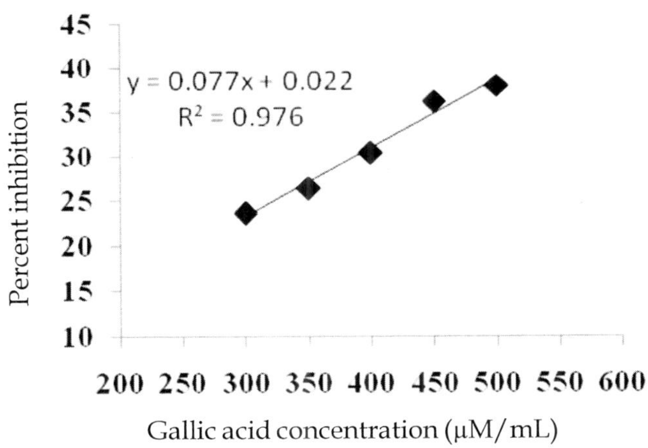

1.2 ABTS (2-2-azinobis-3 ethylbenthiazoline-6-sulphonic acid) radical cation activity

1.2.1 Principle

ABTS is also a relatively stable free radical. This method is based on the ability of antioxidants to quench the long-lived ABTS radical cation, a blue/green chromophore with characteristic absorption at 734 nm, in comparison to that of standard antioxidants (Shirwaikar *et al.*, 2006).

1.2.2 Apparatus and chemicals

- ABTS reagent
- 2.45 mM potassium persulphate
- ABTS Stock solution: Prepare 7 mM ABTS solution using 2.45 mM potassium persulphate ($K_2S_2O_8$) solution and then allow the mixture to stand in the dark at ambient temperature for 16 h. $ABTS^+$ and potassium persulphate react stoichiometrically at a ratio of 1:0.5 (mol/mol). This results in complete oxidation of $ABTS^+$. Oxidation of $ABTS^+$ commenced immediately, but the absorbance was not maximal and stable until 6 h had elapsed. The radical was stable in this form more than two days, when stored in dark at ambient temperature.
- ABTS working solution: Working solution prepared by diluting the stock solution with ethanol to an absorbance of 0.70 at t_0 (t=0 min) and equilibrated at 30°C exactly 6 min after initial mixing.
- Ethanol
- Gallic acid standard
- Whatman filter paper No 42
- Spectrophotometer

1.2.3 Procedure

- Weigh 5g of meat products and triturate with 20 ml of ethanol for 2 min.
- Transfer the content quantitatively into a beaker and filter through Whatman filter paper No 42.
- Take 1 ml of the filtrate in a test tube and mix properly with 2 ml of $ABTS^+$ working standard solution.
- Keep tubes at room temperature under dark for 20 min.
- Take absorbency (t_{20}) at 734 nm.

Calculation

$$ABTS^+ \text{ activity (\% inhibition)} = [(0.7 - At_{20})/0.7] \times 100$$

- Prepare standard calibration curve using different concentration of gallic acid (50-400 μM/ml) and express the result of $ABTS^+$ activity as mg GAE/g of products after comparing with the standard curve.

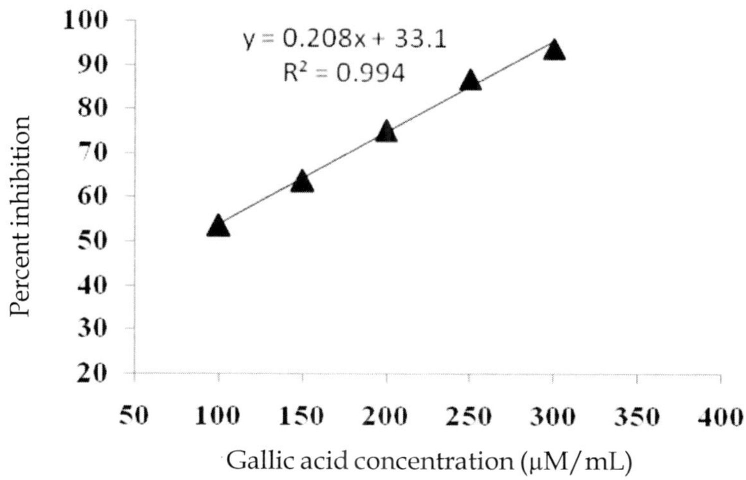

1.3 Superoxide anion scavenging activity (SASA)

1.3.1 Principle

Superoxide anion scavenging activity is determined based on the reduction of nitro-blue- tetrazolium (NBT) in the presence of NADH and phenozonium methosulphate (PMS) under aerobic condition (Kumar and Chattopadhyay, 2007).

1.3.2 Apparatus and chemicals

- 100 μM NBT
- 100 μM NADH
- 100 μM PMS
- 0.2M Tris-HCl buffer (pH 8.0)
- Ethanol
- Gallic acid standard
- Whatman filter paper No 42
- Spectrophotometer

1.3.3 Procedure

- Weigh 5g of meat products and triturate with 20 ml of ethanol for 2 min.
- Transfer the content quantitatively into a beaker and filter through Whatman filter paper No 42.
- Take 150µl NBT (100µM), 450µl NADH (100µM) with 400 µl sample extract in a tube.
- Make up volume to 1 ml with distilled water and then add 1.9 ml of Tris-HCl buffer (0.02M, pH 8.0).
- Add 100 µl of PMS (100 µM, keep the tube under aerobic condition, and finally take absorbance at 560 nm after 20 min.
- Make a blank without the extract.

Calculation

Superoxide anion scavenging activity (%) = [(Absorbance of $_{\text{Blank}}$ – Absorbance of Sample)/ Absorbance $_{\text{Blank}}$] ×100.

- Gallic acid (30-90µM/mL) was used as standard antioxidant.

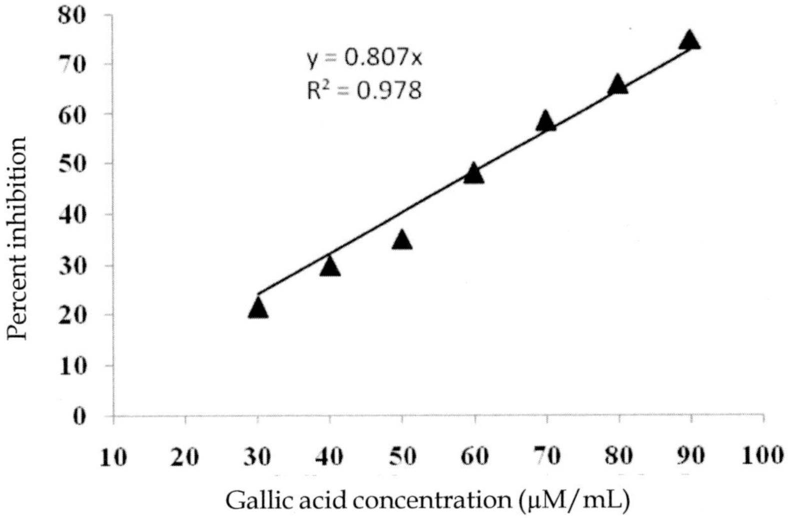

2. Bioactive compound

2.1 Total phenolics

2.1.1 Principle

Determination of total phenolic is important since it indirectly inform the antioxidant potential of a particular functional food product including meat product. Total phenolics can be measured by Folin-Ciocalteau's method and expressed as Gallic acid equivalents (Yuan *et al.,* 2005).

2.1.2 Apparatus and chemicals

- 2.0% Na_2CO_3
- 100 μM NADH
- 100 μM PMS
- 0.2M Tris-HCl buffer (pH 8.0)
- Ethanol
- Gallic acid standard
- Whatman filter paper No 42
- Spectrophotometer

2.1.3 Procedure

- Weigh 5g of meat products and triturate with 20 ml of ethanol for 2 min.
- Transfer the content quantitatively into a beaker and filter through Whatman filter paper No 42.
- Take 100μl of sample extract in a tube, add 2 ml of 2.0% $Na_2CO_{3,}$ mix well and then wait for 2 min.
- Make up volume to 2.4 ml with distilled water.
- Add 100 μl of 1 N Folin-Ciocalteau's reagents and then further incubate at ambient temperature for 30 min.
- Read the absorbance at 720 nm.
- Make a blank without the extract.

Calculation

- Determine the amount of total phenolics using external standard method substituting respective absorbance in the linear regression formula [y = 9207x + 241.55 and R^2 = 0.9949; Where, y = gallic acid concentration, x = absorbance or (sample reading - blank reading) and R^2 = correlation coefficient] after calibration of standard curve of pure gallic acid.

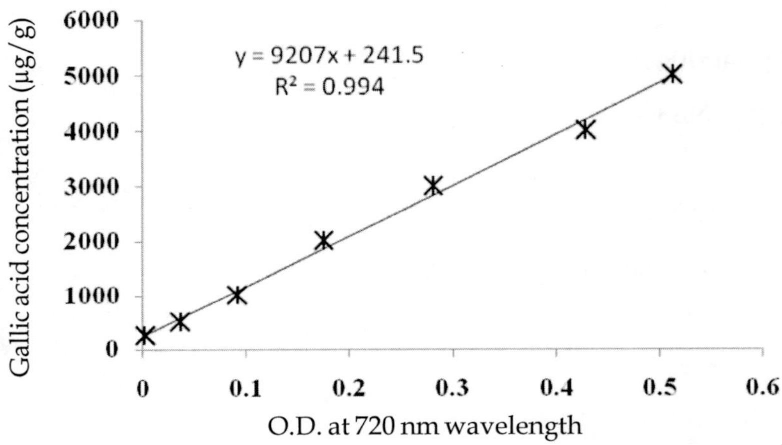

2.2 Total flavonoids

2.2.1 Principle

The flavonoid compounds are extracted with ethanol and when react with the $AlCl_3$ produce colour compounds which are determined by spectrophotometrically (Earnsworth *et al.*, 1974).

2.2.2 Apparatus and chemicals

- 2 % $AlCl_3$
- Gallic acid
- UV-Vis spectrophotometer.

2.2.3 Procedure

- Take 0.5 ml of sample extract and transfer to a test tube containing 0.5 ml of 2 % $AlCl_3$.
- Incubate the tube at 27°C for 1.5 h.

- Take absorbance in a UV-Vis spectrophotometer at 420 nm wavelengths.

Calculation

Calculate the total flavonoids content after calibration of standard curve using gallic acid and express as gallic acid equivalent (GAE, µg/g).

2.3 Gallic acid

2.3.1 Principle

Gallic acid is a water soluble antioxidant compound has greater role in anti-oxidative activity of muscle foods. The Folin-Ciocalteau's method described by Gonzalez *et al.* (2003) can easily apply for determination of gallic acid content.

2.3.2 Apparatus and chemicals

- 15 % Na_2CO_3
- F-C reagent
- Gallic acid
- UV-Vis spectrophotometer

2.3.3 Procedure

- Take 200 µl sample extract
- Mix with reaction mixture containing 2 ml of 15 % Na_2CO_3 solution and 0.5 ml of F-C reagent
- Add 2.3 ml distilled water to make volume up to 5 ml.
- Mix the contents properly, hold for two min and then heat at 50°C for 5 min.
- Cool the tubes to room temperature and read absorbances at 765 nm.

Calculation

Calculate the gallic content after calibration of standard curve using gallic acid and express as gallic acid equivalent (GAE, µg/g).

2.4 Reutin

For the determination of reutin content, method described by Kreft *et al.* (2002) can be followed.

2.4.1 Apparatus and chemicals

- Methanol
- Acetic acid
- Distilled water
- 5 % AlC_3
- Reutin.

2.4.2 Procedure

- Take 0.5 ml of extract and dilute to 10 folds with solvent containing methanol - acetic acid - water (100:2:100; v/v/v).
- Take 2 ml of this diluted solution to a test tube and then mix with 0.2 ml of 5 % AlC_3 in methanol or pure methanol (blank).
- Incubate the reaction tubes at 27 ± 2°C for 30 min under dark.
- Read the absorbance at 420 nm.

Calculation

Calculate the reutin content after calibration of standard curve using gallic acid and express as gallic acid equivalent (GAE, μg/g).

3. Vitamins

3.1 β-carotene

3.1.1 Principle

A simple procedure as developed by Biswas *et al.* (2011) can be followed for determination of total β-carotene cotent from meat produtcs. The β-carotene can be extracted easily from sample matrix with acetone as an extractant and then determine spectrometrically at 449nm wavelength. The amount of β-carotene is calculated after preparation of standard calibration curve and express as mg/g of sample.

3.1.2 Apparatus and chemicals

- Acetone
- β-carotene standard
- Polypropylene centrifuge tube
- Spectrophotometer

3.1.3 Procedure

- Accurately weigh 5 g of sample
- Homogenize with 25 ml of chilled acetone.
- Transfer quantitatively into a polypropylene centrifuge tube, hold at 4 ±1°C for 15 min with occasional shaking, and finally centrifuge at 3,000 rpm for 10 min.
- Collect the supernatant into a separate test tube.
- Re-extract the compound with 25 ml of acetone followed by centrifugation once again as above.
- Combine both of the supernatants and then filter through the Whatman filter paper No. 42.
- Determine the absorbance of the extract at 449 nm wavelength in a UV-Vis spectrophotometer.
- Calculate the amount of β-carotene after calibration of linear standard graph and express as µg/g of sample.

3.2 α-tocopherol acetate (Vitamin E)

The α-tocopherol acetate (Vitamin E) can be measured effectively adopting simple method as reported by Prieto *et al.* (1999) with modification.

3.2.1 Apparatus and chemicals

- 0.6 M sulfuric acid
- 28 mM sodium phosphate
- 4 mM ammonium molybdate
- Vitamin E standard (α-tocopherol acetate)

3.2.2 Procedure

- Take 200 µl of sample extract and transfer in to a test tube containing 2.0 ml of reagent solution (0.6 M sulfuric acid, 28 mM sodium phosphate, and 4 mM ammonium molybdate)
- Incubate at 37°C for 1.5 h with occasional shaking and mixing.
- Measure absorbance of the aqueous phase at 695 nm against the blank.
- The blank prepare using 1 ml of reagent solution and 200 µl of extraction buffer.

Calculation

- Determine the vitamin E (α-tocopherol acetate) content after calibration of standard curve (y = 0.236x + 0.012 and R^2=0.98) using working standard solution and express as µg/ g of sample.

3.3 Ascorbic acid (Vitamin C) (Shrivas et al., 2005)

3.3.1 Principle

Ascorbic acid is oxidized to dehydroascorbic acid which then reacts with 2, 4-dinitro phenylhydrazine, which is dissolved in the sulphuric acid and absorption manimum is read at 500-520 nm.

3.3.2 Apparatus and chemicals

- *Metaphosphoric acetic acid solution:* Dissolve 50 g of metaphosphoric acid, add to it 100 ml of acetic acid and finally make up volume to 1 litre.
- *2, 4-dinitro phenylhydrazine:* Weigh 2 g of 2, 4-dinitro phenyl hydrazine, dissolve with 100 ml of 9N H_2SO_4 and finally filter and store in brown bottle in refrigerator. Refilter a portion of it before use a clear supernatant.
- *Thiourea solution:* Dissolve 10 g thiourea in 100 ml of 50% ethanol and keep at refrigeration temperature.
- *Cupric sulphate solution:* Dissolve 1.5g of cupric sulphate in water and dilute it to 100 ml.
- *Combined colour reagent:* Prepare fresh on the day of use by mixing 15 ml of 2, 4 DNPH. 20.1 ml of cupric sulphate solution and 30.1 ml of thiourea.

- 85% H_2SO_4:To 30 ml of distilled water add 170 ml of conc. H_2SO_4 mix cool stored in glass Stoppard bottle.
- Standard solution: Prepare fresh stock by dissolve 100 mg. Ascorbic Acid in 100 ml of metaphosphoric acid. Dilute 5 ml of stock to 100 ml. 1 ml of this is equal to 50μg of Ascorbic Acid.

3.3.3 Procedure

- Weigh 10 of sample and homogenize with 100 ml of metaphosphoric acid and filter.
- Pipette 1 ml of extract into small test tubes run the experiment in duplicate.
- To each test tube add 1 ml of metaphosphoric acid except blank, in which 2 ml metaphosphoric acid is taken.
- Add 0.4 ml of freshly prepared colour reagent to each test tube and mix.
- Cool in the ice bath for 5 min.
- Add slowly in mixing 2 ml of ice cold 85% H_2SO_4.
- Let the tubes stand at room temperature for 30 min then mix.
- Read the absorbance at 500 nm against blank.
- Prepare standard calibration curve using standard concentration of 10, 20, 30, 40 and 50 μg and calculate.

References

Biswas A. K., J. Sahoo and M. K. Chatli 2011. *LWT - Food Science and Technology. 44:* 1809 –1813.-9.

Earnsworth, N. R., Berderka, J. P. and Moses, M. (1974): *J Pharm Sci 63*: 457- 459.-12.

González, M., Guzman, B. Rudyk, R., Romano, E. and Molina, M. A. A. 2003 *Latin Am J Pharmacy* 22 (3): 243-248.-14.

Kato, K., Terao, S., Shimamoto, N., & Hirata, M. 1988. *J Medicinal Chem* 31(4): 793-798.

Kreft S., Strukejl, B. Gabericik, A. and Kreft, I. 2002. *J Exper Botany* 53: 1801-1804.-21.

Kumar, A. and Chattopadhyay, S. (2007). Food Chemistry, 100(4): 1377-1384.

Prieto, P., M. Pineda and M. Aguilar 1999. *Anal Biochem* 269(2): 337-341.-30.

Shirwaikar, A., Rajendran, K., & Punitha, I. S. R. (2006). *Biological & Pharmaceutical Bulletin*, 29(9): 1906-1910.

Shrivas, K., K. Agrawal and D. K. Patel 2005. *J Chinese Chemical Society* 52: 503-506.-32.

Yuan, Y.V., Bone, D. E. and Carrington, M. F. 2005. *Food Chem* 91(3): 485–494.-39.

□□□

Chapter VII

Techniques for Detection of Tenderizing Enzymes in Meat

1. µ- and m- calpains (Casein zymography method) (Biswas et al., 2016)

Calpains, the calcium-dependent thiol proteases are widely expressed with ubiquitous and tissue specific isoforms and have been implicated in various important cellular processes including cell motility, signal transduction pathways, apoptosis, cell differentiation and regulation of the cytoskeleton through modifying the primary and secondary structural features of target proteins. Therefore, identification of these components in tissue system is frequently important.

1.1 Principle

Zymography is a fascinating technique in molecular biology especially in protein chemistry for measuring non-denatured enzyme activity. In casein zymography proteins are separated by electrophoretic technique under denaturing, non-reducing conditions. It is then allowed to renature and consume the substrate. The separation occurs in a polyacrylamide gel containing a specific substrate that is co-polymerized with the acrylamide. In the casein gels, calpain lyses the protein molecules and thus visualized as clear bands against blue background when stain with a Coomassie Blue R-250 stain.

1.2 Apparatus and reagents

- Mini-Protean Tetra cell system along with accessories (Spacer plate, short plate, casting frame, casting stand, buffer dam, electrophoresis module, companion assembly and mini tank and lid)
- Power pack basic power supply.
- Extraction buffer solution: 50 mM tris – base, (pH 8.3), 10 mM Ethylenediaminetetraacetic acid (EDTA) and 2-Mercaptoethanol. Add 50 μL of 2-Mercaptoethanol per 100 mL (v/v) of 1X solution prepared using Tris-base and EDTA. Add cocktail mixture of protease inhibitors (PMSF, Leupeptin and Ovomucoid) during preparation of meat homogenate for extraction of calpains and calpastatin.
- 6 N HCl, 100 mM PMSF, Leupeptin (5 mg/mL Stock solution), Ovomucoid (300 mg/mL, Stock solution).
- Resolving gel buffer- 1.5 M Tris–base, pH 8.8.
- Stacking gel buffer- 1.32 M Tris–base, pH 6.8.
- Acrylamide/bis–acrylamide stock solution (4:0.16).
- 10 % ammonium persulfate (w/v).
- N, N, N, N 2 -Tetramethyl-ethylenediamine (TEMED).
- Casein purified.
- Sample buffer (3:1, v/v).
- Electrode running buffer (10x, pH8.3): 25 mM Tris–base, pH 8.3 (30.3 g/L), 192 mM glycine (144 g/L), 1 mM EGTA (3.804 g/L), EDTA (3.72 g/L), MCE (500 μL/L, at last after dilution to 1X) .
- Proteolytic buffer (10X, pH 7.4): 20 mM Tris–base (2.42 g/ 100mL), 10 mM DTT (1.54 g/100mL), 4 mM $CaCl_2$ (0.44g/100 mL. Store at 4±1°C.
- Coomassie Brilliant Blue G-250 solution: Dissolve 0.20 g CBB in solution containing 40 mL methanol, 10 mL glacial acetic acid and 50 mL distilled water.
- Destaining solution: Add 30 mL methanol and 10 mL glacial acetic acid in 60 mL distilled water.

1.3 Procedure

- Carry out all the procedures at AC room to avoid denaturation of proteins/enzymes.
- Weigh 0.3 g of finely cut tissue sample; homogenize with 6 volumes of ice-cooled extraction buffer (1.8 mL, pH 8.3) containing 50 mM tris HCl, 10 mM EDTA, 0.05% 2-mercapto-ethanol (MCE).
- Add protease inhibitors (195 μL/10 mL of 100 mM PMSF, 66 μL/10 mL of 300 mg/mL ovomucoid, 12 μL of 5 mg/mL leupeptin) while mixing extraction buffer to prepare homogenate to stop functioning of unwanted proteins/enzymes.
- Centrifuge the content at 12000 rpm for 20 min at 4°C, collect the supernatant in a separate centrifuge tube and disposed-off the sediments.
- Centrifuge the supernatant once again as mentioned earlier and finally load in the gel for casein zymography study.
- Prepare resolving gel using 4.9 mL distilled water, 2.5 mL 1.5 M Tris – base pH 8.8), 2.5 mL Acrylamide/bis–acrylamide (4:0.16), 0.21 mg casein, 40 μL of 10 % APS solution and 28 μL of TEMED. Mix the content.
- Caste the gel in a gel cassette fitted with the casting stand. Allow space for staking gel after placing a comb completely into the assembled gel cassette and marking the glass plate 1 cm below the comb teeth. Remove the comb, pour the resolving gel solution gently using disposable plastic pipette up to the mark, and finally, overlay with t-amyl alcohol or water.
- Allow the gel to polymerize for 1 hour. Rinse the gel surface completely with distilled water. Do not leave the alcohol overlay more than 1h since it will dehydrate the top of the gel.
- Prepare the stacking gel monomer solution using 6.5 mL distilled water, 1 mL Acrylamide/bis–acrylamide (40:1.6) solution and 2.5 mL 1.32 M Tris–bases (pH 6.8). Add 50 μL of 10 % APS solution and 10 μL of TEMED.
- Dry the top of the resolving gel with Whatman filter paper, pour the solution carefully until the top of the short plate and then place 10-wells comb between the spacers. Wait for polymerization.

- Set the clamping frame to the open position on a clean flat surface. Place the first gel cassette with the short plate facing inward on to the gel supports, gel supports are moulded into the bottom of the clamping frame assembly. The gel will now rest at a 30° angle, tilting away from the centre of the clamping frame. Similarly place the second gel on the other side of the clamping frame.
- Place and lock the gel cassettes gently, and if use odd number please you should use buffer dam.
- Fill the assembly upper chamber with buffer to just under the edge of the outer gel plate. Load the samples into the assemblies while they are sitting on a flat surface, in the tank.
- For loading the sample extract mix with the sample buffer (3:1, v/v).
- Load the sample on the casein gel and run the electrophoresis unit at 100 V for 3- 4 h at 4°C in 1X electrode running buffer.
- After end of the electrophoresis, turn off the power supply and disconnect the electrical lead. Remove the tank lid and carefully lift out the electrode assemblies. Pour off and discard the running buffer. Open the arms of the assembly and remove the gel cassettes by gently separating the two plates.
- Incubate the gel in 1X proteolytic buffer for 18 – 24 h at 20°C. In the region of presence of activated calpain, the casein digests into small fragments that diffuse out of the gel.
- Stain the gel with Coomassie Brilliant Blue G-250 for 30 min and then de-stain using destaing solution.
- Presence of clear bands indicates activity of μ - and *m*- calpains.
- The bands now photograph using high resolution camera or using Gel-Doc.

2. Calpains and calpastatin

2.1 SDS-PAGE method

2.1.1 Principle

Calpastatin does not have proteolytic domain for its activity but it acts through inhibitory activity of calpains, so its identification using

SDS-PAGE is important. SDS-PAGE also visualizes different domain structure of both μ- and m-calpains in the sample.

2.1.2 Apparatus and chemicals

- Analytical grade chemicals, reagents and solvents and protease inhibitors of high purity are required to complete this experiment. Prepare all solutions using deionised water and store in chilled condition until further use.
- Muscle samples required for the experiment should collect immediately after slaughter and transfer in to a self-sealing LDPE bags.
- Blood samples (15 mL) should collect suitable means (Jugular / Wing vein) or during bleeding operations. Collect the samples in vials containing EDTA (1 mg/mL blood) and transfer to the laboratory for processing immediately.
- *Preparation of tissue homogenate:* Always collect fresh tissue samples immediately after slaughter to avoid autolytic degradation or denaturation of calpains and calpastatin. Prepare the sample extract in chilled condition or hold the tissues at -20°C until use. Procedure for preparation of tissue homogenate is similar to that mention for sample extraction protocol for casein Zymography.
- Mini-Protean Tetra cell system along with accessories (Spacer plate, short plate, casting frame, casting stand, buffer dam, electrophoresis module, companion assembly and mini tank and lid).
- Power pack basic power supply.
- *Dialysis buffer (pH 7.4):* Dialysis buffer contains 40 mM Tris-base, 5 mM EDTA and 0.05% 2-MCE. For working dialysis buffer solution take 100 mL each 40 mM Tris-base and 5 mM EDTA solution in a graduated beaker, add deionized water to about 900 mL volume, adjust pH to 7.4 and finally transfer in to a measuring cylinder to make up volume to 1000 mL. Add 500 µL 2-mercapto-ethanol. Hold at refrigeration temperature until further use. Use fresh dialysis buffer each time.
- *Equilibration buffer (pH 7.4):* Equilibration buffer contains 40 mM Tris-base, 0.5 mM EDTA and 0.05 % 2-MCE. For preparation of

working solution take 10 mL each 40 mM Tris-base and 0.5 mM EDTA solution in a graduated beaker, add deionized water to about 95 mL volume, adjust pH to 7.4 and finally transfer in to a measuring cylinder to make up volume to 100 mL. Add 50μL 2-mercaptoethanol and 50 mg of sodium azide (NaN_3). Hold at refrigeration temperature until further use.

- *Eluting buffer:* Prepare eluting buffers of various concentrations of NaCl in equilibration buffer.
  - *100 mM NaCl*: Take 0.584 g of NaCl in a graduated beaker and dissolve with equilibration buffer to about the volume of100 mL. Store at refrigeration temperature.
  - *200 mM NaCl*: Weigh 1.169 g of NaCl, transfer to a graduated glass beaker and make up the volume as mention for preparation of 100 mM concentration of NaCl.
  - *400 mM NaCl*: Accurately weigh 2.337 g of NaCl, transfer to a measuring cylinder and make up volume to 100 mL using equilibration buffer. Transfer to a conical flask and store at 4°C.
  - *2 M NaCl*: Weigh 11.68 g NaCl in a graduated beaker, add equilibration buffer to about 95 mL volume, mix well and finally transfer in to a measuring cylinder to make up volume to 100 mL. Transfer to a conical flask and hold at refrigeration temperature until further use.
- *Anion exchange column (DEAE Sephacel)*: Anion exchanger is use for packing the column. Use Pasteur pipette to draw swollen DEAE sephacel matrix and pour carefully without touching the sidewall of the column. Pack a column (1.77 cm inner dimension) with the matrix to about 5 cm length and wait for 40 – 50 min to settle down properly.
- *Resolving gel buffer*- 1.5 M Tris–base, pH 8.8.
- *Stacking gel buffer*- 1.32 M Tris–base, pH 6.8.
- *Acrylamide/bis–acrylamide stock solution* (40:1.6).
- *10% (w/v) SDS buffer.*
- *10 % ammonium persulfate (w/v).*
- *N, N, N, N* 2 *-Tetramethyl-ethylenediamine (TEMED).*

- *0.5% (w/v) Bromophenol blue.*
- *Sample buffer* (1:2, v/v): For preparation of 10 mL sample buffer, add 3.55 mL deionised water, 1.25 mL1.32M tris-base (pH 6.8), 2.5 mL glycerol, 2 mL 10 % (v/v) SDS and 0.2 mL 0.5% (w/v) Bromophenol Blue. Mix well and finally add 50 µL 2- MCE just before use.
- *Electrode running buffer* (10x, pH8.3): 25 mM Tris–base, pH 8.3 (30.3 g/L), 192 mM glycine (144 g/L), 1 % (10 g/ L). For use, dilute 50 mL of 10X stock solution with 450 mL deionised water for each electrophoresis run.
- *Coomassie Brilliant Blue G-250 solution*: Dissolve 0.20 g CBB in solution containing 40 mL methanol, 10 mL glacial acetic acid and 50 mL distilled water.
- *Destaining solution*: Add 40 methanol and 10 glacial acetic acid in 50 mL distilled water.

2.1.3 Procedure

- Put supernatant prepared earlier into dialysis a tube (12 kDa MWCO) for overnight at 4°C in dialysis buffer containing 40 mM tris-base, 5 mM EDTA and 0.05 % 2-mercaptoethanol (pH 7.4).
- Open one end of dialysis tube and transfer into a centrifuge tube.
- Centrifuge the solution at 7000 rpm for 10 min at 4 °C.
- The supernatant equivalent to 5 g of meat sample load on 1.5 cm × 5 cm DEAE Sephacel column (anion exchanger) equilibrated with 3 washings of 20 ml equilibration buffer containing 40 mM tris-base, 0.5 mM EDTA and 0.05% 2-mercaptoethanol (pH 7.4).
- Collect 3 fractions of 4 ml each at different concentrations of NaCl.
- Elute calpastatin 100 mM NaCl; μ-calpain at 200 mM NaCl and m-calpain at 400 mM NaCl in equilibration buffer.
- Store all the eluted fractions (4 + 4 + 4 = 12) at -20 °C until load in the SDS-PAGE or biochemical assay for quantification.
- Carry out all the procedures at AC room to avoid denaturation of proteins/enzymes.

- Prepare resolving gel containing 10 % acrylamide (w/v), 0.4% bis-acrylamide (w/v) in 375 mM tris-base (pH 8.8), 0.1% (w/v) SDS, 0.05% (w/v) APS and 0.05% (v/v) TEMED.
- Prepare the stacking gel using 4% acrylamide (w/v), 0.16% bis-acrylamide (w/v) in 330 mM tris-base (pH 6.8), 0.1% (w/v) SDS, 0.05% APS and 0.1% TEMED.
- Dilute the purified fraction at 1:2 ratio with sample buffer containing 66 mM tris-base (pH 6.8), 26 % (v/v) glycerol, 2.1 % (w/v) SDS, 0.01 % (w/v) bromophenol blue and 5 % (v/v) MCE.
- Heat the sample at 95°C for 5 min before loading in the wells.
- Perform gel electrophoresis at constant voltage of 120 V for 90 min with the electrode running buffer containing 192 mM glycine, 25 mM tris-base (pH 8.3) and 0.1 % SDS.
- Load the standard protein ladder (marker) in one of the gel well.
- Upon completion of electrophoresis, stain the gel for 1 h in a solution containing 0.25% Coomassie Brilliant Blue G-250, 40 % methanol and 10 % acetic acid
- De-stained in a solution comprising 40 % (v/v) methanol and 10 % (v/v) acetic acid.
- Identify the bands corresponding to M.Wt. marker and record.

2.2 Biochemical test

Quantification of calpains and calpastatin is important to understand possible effect of these enzymes on post-mortem tenderization of meat. During tenderization process micro-calpain lyses many cytoskeletal proteins also act on some myofibrillar proteins thereby improve tenderness.

2.2.1 Principle

Calpain lyses the protein molecules (casein) in the solution and produce blue chromophore which is measure spectrophotometrically in the presence of Ca^{2+} and EDTA buffer.

2.2.2 Apparatus and reagents

- Spectrophotometer

- Anion exchange column with column matrix (DEAE Sephacel)
- Dialysis buffer (pH 7.4) contains 40 mM Tris-base, 5 mM EDTA and 0.05% 2-MCE: For working solution take 100 mL each 40 mM Tris-base and 5 mM EDTA solution in a graduated beaker, add deionized water to about 900 mL volume, adjust pH to 7.4 and finally transfer in to a measuring cylinder to make up volume to 1000 mL. Add 500 μL 2-mercapto-ethanol. Hold at refrigeration temperature until further use. Use fresh dialysis buffer each time.
- Equilibration buffer (pH 7.4) contains 40 mM Tris-base, 0.5 mM EDTA and 0.05 % 2-MCE. For preparation of working solution take 10 mL each 40 mM Tris-base and 0.5 mM EDTA solution in a graduated beaker, add deionized water to about 95 mL volume, adjust pH to 7.4 and finally transfer in to a measuring cylinder to make up volume to 100 mL. Add 50μL 2-mercaptoethanol and 50 mg of sodium azide (NaN_3). Hold at refrigeration temperature until further use.
- Eluting buffer: Prepare eluting buffers of 100, 200 and 400 mM concentrations of NaCl in equilibration buffer.
- 2 M NaCl buffer.
- 5 mM calcium chloride, 5% trichloroacetic acid,1 mM NaN_3, 5 mg/ml casein, 10 mM 2-mercaptoethanol, 6N Acetic acid,10 mM EDTA.

2.2.3 Procedure

- Pool 0.5 ml aliquot from the each fraction containing μ- and *m*-calpains in separate tubes.
- Add 1.5 ml of assay buffer containing 100 mM tris-base (pH adjusted at 7.5 with 6N Acetic acid), 5 mM $CaCl_2$, 1 mM NaN_3, 5 mg/ml casein and 10 mM 2-mercaptoethanol and incubate for 60 min at 25°C.
- Add 2 ml of 5% trichloroacetic acid (TCA) to terminate the reaction.
- Precipitate the insoluble proteins by centrifugation at 2,000 x *g* for 30 min.
- Measure the soluble proteins of each fraction at A_{278} in Biospectrometer.

- Determine calcium-independent proteolytic activity of each fraction by replacing $CaCl_2$ with 10 mM EDTA in the reaction mixture.
- Take absorbance of the reaction tube at 278 nm weave length to determine Ca^{2+} dependent proteolytic activity.
- Make blanks using 0.5 ml of 200 mM NaCl and 400 mM NaCl in equilibration buffer for μ- and *m*-calpain containing fractions respectively in 1.5 ml of assay buffer containing either $CaCl_2$ or EDTA. (One unit of calpain activity was defined as the amount of enzyme that catalyzed an increase of 1.0 absorbance unit at A_{278} after 60 min at 25°C).
- Measure calpastatin activity by incubating appropriate amounts of pooled fractions containing calpastatin and *m*-calpain at 4°C for 1 min before adding 1.5 ml assay buffer containing $CaCl_2$ to start the reaction.
- Terminate the reaction by adding 2 ml 5 % TCA and centrifuged as before.
- Take three tubes assay inhibitor activity: (1) *m*-calpain pooled fraction (0.5 ml), incubated with assay buffer containing $CaCl_2$; (2) *m*-calpain (0.5 ml) plus calpastatin (0.5 ml), incubated in assay buffer as described in 1; (3) calpastatin alone, incubated in assay buffer containing EDTA (One unit of calpastatin activity is defined as the amount of calpastatin that inhibits one unit of *m*-calpain).

Calculation

- Calculate the total activity of **micro or milli calpain** by multiplying Ca^{2+}-dependent proteolytic activity by the dilution factor.

CDP Activity (Units/g) = ($A_{278}CaCl_2$ buffer A_{278} EDTA buffer) x dilution factor.

- Calculate total inhibitory activity by the calpastatin as-

  Total inhibitor activity = 1 – (2 – 3) × dilution factors.

Notes:

1. Dilution factor is calculated by volumes of extraction buffer + elution buffer used per g of muscle sample before analysis. If total volume is 18 mL for per g then dilution factor will be 18.

3. Cathepsin B, D and H (Jamadar and Harikumar, 2002)

The cathepsins are proteolytic enzymes have important role in post-mortem tenderization of meat in particularly when the pH of meat is achieved below 6.0. The cathepsin group of enzymes show best activity at pH lower than ultimate pH of meat (5.4-5.6). So activity determination of these enzymes in meat system may predict possible cathepsin induced post-mortem tenderness of meat.

3.1 Apparatus and chemicals

- 0.1 M acetate buffers (pH 3.8).
- 1 % haemoglobin (prepared in 0.1 M acetate buffer).
- 10 % trichloroacetic acid.
- Nα - benzoyl - DL - arginine β-napthylamide (BANA), pH 6.2 & 6.8.
- Pestle and mortar, test tubes.

3.2 Procedure

Cathepsin D

- Weigh 10 g tissue sample and homogenize with 100 mL of 0.1 M acetate buffers (pH 3.8).
- Take 200 μL of meat homogenate and then add 500 μL acetate buffer and 1.0% haemoglobin.
- Hold the tube at 50°C for 30 min and then add 1 mL 10 % TCA solution to terminate the reaction.
- The TCA soluble products are determined using tyrosine as a standard.

Cathepsin B

- The activity of cathepsin B is determined using BANA at pH 6.2 at 40°C for 1 h and the reaction is terminated using 1 mL mersayl acid.

Cathepsin H

- The activity of cathepsin H is determined using BANA at pH 6.8 at 40°C for 30 min and the reaction is terminated by adding 1 mL mersayl acid.

- The activity is determined by monitoring the release of β–naphthylamine at 520 nm and expressed as mM/h/g tissue.

4. ATPase activity

4.1 Principle

ATP is the source of energy for muscle contraction, for pumping of calcium during relaxation, and for maintaining the sodium and potassium gradients across the sarcolema. This energy is derived form a reaction, catalysed by the ATPase, in which ATP is hydrolysed to ADP and inorganic phosphate. ATPase activity proceeds at a slow rate during low temperature storage of meat. The estimation of ATPase gives an idea about the extent of breakdown of ATP and progress of rigor mortis.

4.2 Equipment

Fine analytical balance, high speed blender (15000 rpm), Spectrophotometer.

4.3 Reagents

- Reaction mixture- consist of 1 M NaCl- 1.2 ml (120mm), 1M KCl- 0.30 ml (30 mm), 1M MgCl2- 0.05 ml (5 mm) , bovine serum albumin 0.2 %- 0.1 ml and 3.35 ml glass distilled water. Use 0.25 ml per assay for a final volume of 0.5 ml, (pH 7.4 at 37^{0}C).
- 30 mm ATP- dissolve 181.8 mg (disodium salt) in 6 ml water, adjust pH with 0.5 M tris base and make upto 10 ml with glass distilled water, store in freezer.
- 50 % TCA (W/W) in water.

Procedure

- Meat homogenate – homogenise one gram of meat sample with 10 ml of ice cold water in a vortex mixer and filter through cotton gauge to remove fascia.
- Estimate protein content of homogenate by Lowry's method or Biuret method.
- Take 0.25 ml reaction mixture in two test tubes.

- Add 0.05 ml homogenate to both the tubes.
- Make the volume of incubation mixture to 0.45 ml with glass distilled water.
- Start reaction at 37^{0}C with the addition of 0.05 ml of ATP solution.
- Stop the reaction after 10 minutes by adding 0.05 ml of 50% TCA and immerse the tubes in ice bath for 10 minutes.
- Run a blank in similar way but the enzyme is added after addition of TCA.
- Centrifuge the tubes for 5 minutes at 5000 rpm to remove precipitate.
- Use the entire supernatant for inorganic phosphate (pi) assay by the method of Fiske and Suba Rao (1967).

Calculation

The enzyme activity is expressed as m moles of pi liberated/hr/ mg protein.

OD unknown/OD standard x concentration standard/mg of protein x 2.

References

Biswas AK, Tandon S, Beura C K 2016. *Food Chem* 200: 315-321.

Fiske and Suba Rao, 1967. *Life science* 6, 595.

Jamadar, S.N. and Harikumar, P. 2002. *J. Food Technol.* 39(1): 72–73.

Paul Ottolenghue, 1975. *Biochem J.* 151, 61-6.

❑❑❑

Chapter VIII

Methods for Monitoring of Food Additives and Chemical Residues

1. Chemical method for identification of important food additives

The nitrate/nitrite is generally used in meat products to stabilize colour of the lean tissue, characteristic flavour of cured meat, inhibit the growth of a numbers of food poisoning and food spoilage microorganisms and to retard development of rancidity. Nitrate is not generally under use at the present day except some specialty items like country cured hams and Lebanon bologna as it takes some times to convert into nitrite before its action. Sodium nitrite is considered most useful additives in the manufacture of cured meat products and present day without such ingredient products rarely comes in the market. Sodium nitrite is the primary ingredient used to produce the heat stable cure colour development (nitrosylhemochromogen). However, some controversies arising with the use of nitrite, as the reaction of nitrous acid with secondary amines produce nitrosamines which shown to have carcinogenic effect to humans. Formation of N-nitrosopyrrolidine during frying of bacon has been major problem from nitrosamines in processed meat.

1.1 Nitrate (Xylenol method)

1.1.1 Principle

The hot water extract of sample react with the m-Xylenol, formed colour compounds which is measured spectrophotometrically, and determined with the comparison of corresponding values of known standard after calibration of standard curve.

1.1.2 Chemicals and materials

- Meta-Xylenol, 1-hydroxy-2, 4-Dimethyl benzene.
- Silver sulphate (Nitrate free).
- Potassium permanganate.
- Ammonium hydroxide.
- Phosphotungstic acid.
- H_2SO_4.
- Sodium hydroxide pellets.
- Sodium nitrate.
- Silver-ammonium hydroxide solution-Dissolve 5 g of nitrate free silver sulphate in 60 mL NH_4OH. Heat to boiling point, concentrate to about 30 mL, cool and dilute to 100 ml with water.
- Bromocresol green indicator: Dissolve 0.1 g bromocresol green in 1.5 mL 0.1 N NaOH and dilute to 100 mL with water.
- Nitrate standard solution: Dissolve 0.181 g recrystalised KNO_3 in water and dilute to 1 litre or dilute 17.85 mL 0.1 N HNO_3 to 1 litre, 10 mL contains 0.25 mg nitrate.
- Sulphuric acid solution: 1 parts of sulphuric acid plus 10 parts of distilled water (v/v).
- Sulphuric acid solution: 3 parts of sulphuric acid plus 1 parts of distilled water (v/v).
- 0.2 N Potassium permanganate solution.
- Phosphotungstic acid solution: 20 g in 100 mL.
- Sodium hydroxide solution: 10 g NaOH in 1 Lit distilled water.

1.1.3 Procedure

- Take accurately 10 g finely minced sample in a beaker and mixed with 80 mL warm water. Then heat on steam bath for 1 h with stirring occasionally.
- Cool to room temperature, transfer to a volumetric flask and finally make volume up to 100 mL. Filter it, and take 25 mL filtrate in 50 mL volumetric flask.

- Add 3 drops bromocresol green indicator and diluted H_2SO_4 solution (1:10) drop-wise until colour changes to yellow.
- Add 0.2 N $KMNO_4$ solution drop-wise with shaking until faint pink remains about 1 minute.
- Add 1 mL H_2SO_4 (3:1) and 1 mL phosphotungstic acid solution.
- Dilute to volume 50 mL with water, mix and filter.
- Transfer 20 mL of aliquot to a 500 mL Erlenmeyer flask containing 0.025 to 0.25 mg $NaNO_3$.
- Add sufficient silver-ammonium hydroxide solution (2 mL) to precipitate chlorides and most of excess phosphotungstic acid.
- Add H_2SO_4 solution (3:1) about 3 times volume of liquid in flask.
- Stopper the flask, mix, cool to about 35°C and add 0.05 mL of the m-Xylenol, stopper, shake and held 30 min at 30 – 40°C (Yellow to brownish yellow colour, indicative of nitrates, appears.
- Bright red precipitate, due to incomplete phosphotungstic acid may also appear.
- Slight excess of phosphotungstic acid possess no interference but large excess may do so.
- After nitration is complete, add 150 mL water, taking care to wash off stopper, and distill 40 - 50 mL into receiver containing 5 mL NaOH.
- Quickly remove any nitroxylenol solidifying in condensor by stopping water flow and letting condensor becomes warm. Transfer 50 mL distillate to 100 mL volumetric flask.
- Dilute to volume with water, and determine $NaNO_3$ by comparing reading of colour of suitable aliquot with standard curve prepared at about 450 nm using water as blank.
- Prepare colour standard from 10 mL nitrate standard solution, using 0.05 ml m-Xylenol and 30 mL H_2SO_4 (3:1) and dilute distillate to 500 mL.

Calculation

$$\text{Sodium nitrate (\%)} = \frac{20A}{B \times C} - 1.232D$$

A = $NaNO_3$ content (mg) in the solution as read from the standard curve.

B = Sample weight in g

C = Aliquot used for nitration

D = % sodium nitrite determined.

Notes:

- For standard curve preparation transfer 0, 0.025, 0.05, 0.1, 0.2 and so on up to 10 mL of standard nitrate solution (0.2 g made to 1 Lit) in to a series of 500 mL Erlenmeyer flask and add 10 mL distilled water in each flask.
- Add 30 mL H_2SO_4 solution (3:1) in each flask, mix, cool to about 35 °C and add 0.05 mL of the m-Xylenol, stopper, shake and held 30 min at 30-40 °C (Yellow to brownish yellow colour, indicative of nitrates, appears).
- Add 150 mL water taking care to wash off the stopper.
- Distill 40-50 mL in from each flask using Kjeldahl assembly into 100 mL graduated measuring cylinder containing 5 mL NaOH.
- Transfer 50 mL distillate to 100 mL volumetric flask.
- Make up volume with water, and read at 450 nm using water as blank.

1.2 Nitrites

1.2.1 Principle

The aqueous extract of sample react with the GRIESS reagent (sulphanilic acid and α-naphthylamine HCl) formed colour compounds which is measured spectrophotometrically, and determined with the comparison of corresponding values of known standard after calibration of standard curve.

1.2.2 Chemicals and materials

- α-naphthylamine HCl.
- Sulphanilic acid.

- Glacial acetic acid.
- Sodium nitrite.
- Hydrochloric acid.
- Mercuric chloride.
- Sulphanilic acid solution-Dissolve 0.5 g of sulphanilic acid in 150 mL of 15 % acetic acid (v/v).
- α-naphthylamine HCl solution: Boil 0.1 g of the chemical in 20 mL water until dissolved and pour hot into 150 mL of 15 % acetic acid.
- Mix solution of (1) and (2) and store tightly closed amber colour glass bottle at refrigeration temperature. This is modified griess reagent.
- Standard solution of nitrite (5µg/mL).
- Mercuric chloride solution (saturated): Add about 70 g of mercuric chloride in 1 Lit of water at 20°C.

1.2.3 Procedure

- Accurately weigh 5.0 g finely minced meat and place in 250 mL volumetric flask. Add 100 mL distilled water and mix properly with glass rod.
- Heat the mixture to 80°C in a water bath with continuous breakage of lumps.
- After completion of heating add 5 mL of saturated mercuric chloride solution and mix. Add enough, hot water to bring volume to about 250 mL.
- Cool to room temperature, dilute to volume with nitrite free water and mix again.
- Filter through Whatman No 1 filter paper and transfer 10 mL of filtrate (represent 0.2 g sample) to 50 mL volumetric flask, add 2 mL of griess reagent, mix and let colour develop for 1 h.
- Transfer suitable portion of solution to photometer cell and determine absorbance at 520 nm against blank of 50 mL water 2 mL reagent.

- Determine nitrite present by comparison with standard curve.
- For preparation of standard curve dilute suitable volume standard nitrite solution to volume in 50 ml volumetric flask, add 2 mL reagent and proceed as above.
- Standard curve is straight line to 5 μg sodium nitrite in final solution.

1.3 Salt and chlorides

Salt (NaCl) is basic to all curing mixture and is the only ingredient require for curing of meat. Light sodium salts (food grade) are used curing of meat. Salt use has a limitation in products not to exceed 2.5% of the finished products (BIS Standard). However, use of salt alone gives harsh, dry, salty product with crumbly texture and undesirable colour that is not very palatable, and objectionable by the consumers. Salts also act as prooxidants due to presence of certain metal impurities. To overcome these undesirable effects of salt, it is generally used in combination with sugar and nitrite and/ or nitrate. But some meat cuts are still cured with salt alone, especially fatty cuts that contain lean (fat back, clear plates, jowls, heavy bellies etc) which are intended for seasoning of other food products. Excessive use of NaCl in food leads to increase of hypertension, blood pressure and many other ailments related to heart diseases to human health. So determination of salt and chloride concentration in muscle food is important.

1.3.1 Salt (NaCl) content

1.3.1.1 Principle

The meat sample is digested with nitric acid in the presence of an excess of silver nitrate which is ten titrated with ammonium thiocyanate and the salt calculated from the amount of Ag^+ required to precipitate the Cl^- present in the sample.

1.3.1.2 Apparatus and reagents

- Weighing balance, burette, hot plate, pipette, conical flask, beaker, measuring cylinder, volumetric flask, Erlenmeyer flask etc.
- Sodium chloride, silver nitrate, ammonium thiocyanate, ferric ammonium sulphate, diethyl ether, nitric acid (free of sodium chloride) and potassium permanganate.

- *0.5 N Silver nitrate solution*: Weigh 84.95 g of silver nitrate in a graduated glass beaker, add distilled water to about 950 mL and mix gently. Transfer into a volumetric flask and make up the volume to 1litre. Store in cool place until use.
- *10% Potassium permanganate*: Weigh 10 g potassium permanganate, transfer to a beaker, and finally dissolve with distilled water to about 100 mL. Transfer into a measuring cylinder and make the final volume to 100 mL. The solution qualitatively dispense in to a conical flask, stopper and store in cool place until use.
- *Saturated ferric ammonium sulphate solution*: Measure 95 mL distilled water, acidified with 5 mL nitric acid and then add 139 g of ferric ammonium sulphate. Mix well, transfer to a volumetric flask and store at room temperature. Before using, ensure that all ferric ammonium sulphate dissolve completely in the solution.
- *0.1N Ammonium thiocyanate solution*: Accurately weigh 76.13 g of ammonium thiosulphate, transfer to a graduated beaker, mix well and finally dispense into a volumetric flask. Store in cool place until use.

1.3.1.3 Procedure

- Take 5 g of sample in an Erlenmeyer flask.
- Add 5 mL of 0.5N silver nitrate solution; wait for 5 - 10 min.
- Add 15 mL nitric acid; boil for two min on a hot plate.
- Stop heating when sample dissolve completely.
- Add small portion of 10% potassium permanganate solution, continue to heat until potassium permanganate disappears and solution becomes colourless.
- Add 25 mL distilled water, heat for another 5- 10 min.
- Cool to room temperature, add water to about 150 mL, and finally add 5 mL ferric ammonium sulphate indicator.
- Add 10 mL diethyl-ether and titrate with 0.1 N ammonium-thiocyanate.

Calculation

$$\text{NaCl (\%)} = \frac{\text{(mL of 0.5 N silver nitrate added - 0.2}\times\text{mL of 0.1 N ammonium thiocyanate)}}{\text{Weight of sample}} \times 2.92$$

1.3.2 Chorides content

1.3.2.1 Apparatus and reagents

- Weighing balance, burette, pipette, conical flask, beaker, measuring cylinder, volumetric flask, pH meter etc
- *4N Nitric acid solution*: Add one volume of nitric acid in 3 volume of distilled water.
- *1.0* N NaOH solution.
- Charcoal (activate).
- *0.1 N Potassium thiocyanate solution*: Weigh 9.7 g of potassium thiocyanate in a graduated glass beaker, add distilled water to about 950 mL and mix gently. Transfer into a volumetric flask and make up the volume to 1litre. Store in cool place until use.
- *0.1N Silver nitrate solution*: Weigh 16.99 g oven dried silver nitrate, transfer to a beaker, and finally dissolve with distilled water to about 1000 mL. Transfer into a measuring cylinder and make the final volume to 1000 mL. The solution transfer in to a conical flask, stopper it and then store in cool place until use.
- *Saturated ammonium iron sulphate indicator solution*: Measure 100 mL distilled water, add slowly ammonium iron sulphate and continue to add until dissolve in the solution. The transfer to a volumetric flask and store at room temperature. Before using, ensure that all ammonium iron sulphate dissolve completely in the solution.
- *Potassium ferricyanide solution (Reagent I)*: Accurately weigh 106 g potassium ferricyanide, transfer to a graduated beaker, and add water to about 1000 mL. Mix well and finally transfer into a volumetric flask. Store in cool place until use.
- *Zinc acetate-glacial acetic acid* solution: Weigh 220 g zinc acetate and transfer to a graduated glass beaker. Then measure 30 mL of glacial acetic acid and dispense into the same beaker. Add distilled water to about 1000 mL and mix slowly and gently. Store solution in a cool place.

1.3.2.2 Procedure

- Accurately weigh 10 g of meat sample, transfer to a conical flask, add 0.5 g of activated charcoal, and finally add 100 mL distilled water.
- Heat to boil for 15 min in water bath.
- Cool to room temperature, add 2 mL of reagent I and II each and then adjust pH to about 7.5-8.3 using 1.0 N sodium hydroxide solution.
- Wait for 30-35 min, transfer the content quantitatively into a 200 mL volumetric flask and make up the volume with distilled water.
- Filter the solution through Whatman filter paper No. 1.
- Take 20 mL filtrate in to a conical flask; add 5 mL 4N nitric acid solution and 1 mL saturated ammonium iron sulphate indicator solution.
- Add 20 mL 0.1N silver nitrate solution and 3 mL nitrobenzene.
- Shake the content vigorously, collect the supernatant and titrate with potassium thiocyanate.

Calculation

Chloride content (% of sodium chloride) = 5.8844 (20-V)/Weight of sample

Where,

V = mL of potassium thiocyanate requires for titration.

1.4 Nitrosamines

1.4.1 Background

Sodium nitrite is considered most useful additives in the manufacture of cure meat products. It is used to produce the heat stable cure colour development (nitrosyl hemochromogen). Sodium nitrite, through a series of chemical reactions, react with meat pigment, myoglobin. The haem ring of Mb is the non-protein portion that is directly involved in the cure colour formation. The heme rings contains the sixth co-ordination position associated with the iron atom (Fe) which is the site where oxygen, water, and other reactive ligands can bind and produce acceptable cure colour of the products. However some controversies arising with the use of nitrite, as the reaction of nitrous acid (which formed by the breakdown of nitrite) with secondary amines produce nitrosamines which shown to have carcinogenic effect to humans. Formation of N-nitrosopyrrolidine during frying of bacon has been major problem from nitrosamines in processed meat. But this can be largely eliminated by the using alpha-tocoferol coated salt in the cure. Sodium erythorbate or ascorbic acid can also reduce the formation of N-nitrosamines when added to pickle. Sodum ascorbate at a level of 550 ppm in combination of 120 ppm sodium nitrite will materially reduce the nitrosamines formation in cured, cooked bacon. However, determination of nitrosamines in processed meat products is important for consumer safety and fair trade.

1.4.2 Apparatus and reagents

- N-nitrosodimethylamine, N-nitrosodiethylamine, N-nitrosopiperidine and N-nitrosopyrrolidine, SPME [Fused silica fibres, coated with polydimethylsiloxane-divinylbenzene (PDMS-DVB, 65 μm) and polyacrylate (PA, 85 μm) coated fibers].
- Standard stock solutions of NDMA, NDEA, NPIR and NPYP: Prepare standards with methanol to a final concentration of 1000 μg/L.
- *Working solutions (100 μg/L):* Prepare daily by dilution of the standard stock solution with Milli-Q water.
- Nitrite cured fried meat products.
- *Gas chromatography condition*: An Agilent 6890 gas chromatograph interfaced with a thermal energy analyzer detector (TEA), Model 610 Thermo Orion, operating in the nitrosamine mode. HP-INOWAX mega bore column (30 m × 530 μm ID × 1μm film thickness, from Agilent). The operating conditions require: injector temperature, 200°C; oven temperature at 100 °C for 3 min, then to 140 °C at 40 °C/ min and then to 160 °C at 5 °C min. The TEA furnace and the GC-TEA interface temperatures- 550 and 250 °C, respectively. Carrier gas- helium flow-rate 5 mL/min.

- *HS-SPME – extraction of NDMA, NDEA, NPIR and NPYP in aqueous solution*: Prepare aqueous standard solutions (12 mL), containing 30 μg/L of NDMA, NDEA, NPIP and NPYR in 36 % (m/v) NaCl and pour into a 24 mL headspace vial. Introduce a small stirring bar, place HS vial in a thermostated water bath, stir the solution using magnetic sterrior and after 10 min expose the fiber in the vapor phase above the liquid sample. After that withdraw the fiber into the needle, and then introduce into the injection port of the GC. Perform the desorption procedure of the analyte from the fiber coating at 200 °C for 8 min.
- *HS-SPME – extraction of NDMA, NDEA, NPIR and NPYP in fortified meat products*: About 2.5 g of previous ground and homogenized sample fortify with 360 ng of each nitrosamine. Add the fortified samples to the HS vial and add enough water to make-up the volume to 12 mL. Follow the HS-SPME extraction in the same procedure as described for the aqueous solution.

1.4.3 Procedure

- Place five portions (2.50 g) of the product samples in 24 mL vials sealed with Teflon–silicone septa.
- Add water to a volume of 12 mL.
- In the first sample introduce a small stirring bar and place the HS vial in a thermostated water bath at 45°C.
- Stir the solution using magnetic sterir and after 10 min expose the PDMS-DVB (65 μm) fiber to the vapor phase above the sample.
- After an extraction time of 25 min, withdraw the fiber into the needle.
- Introduce the injection port to the GC.
- Perform the desorption procedure of the analyte from the fiber coating at 200°C for 8 min using the chromatographic conditions described earlier.
- For second sample, spike the sample with 0.6 mL of a working standard solution containing 100 μg/L of NDMA, NDEA, NPIR and NPYP in a HS-vial.
- Follow the treatment according to the procedure previously described for the sample.

- Spike the other three vials with 2.4; 3.6; 4.8 and 7.2 mL, respectively.
- Determine the nitrosamines directly from the chromatogram after calibration of standard curve and express as mg/kg or µg/kg of sample.

1.5 Phosphates and residual phosphates

1.5.1 Phosphates

1.5.1.1 Apparatus and reagents

- Diluted nitric acid
- Quimociac reagent
- Gooch crucible, Glass fibre, filter paper, Steam bath, Oven, Dessicator.

1.5.1.2 Procedure

- Weigh 2.5 g of sample in an ashing dish.
- Dry for 30 minutes at 125°C in a forced -draft oven.
- Ash at 55°C.
- Add 25 ml diluted nitric acid.
- Heat on steam bath for 30 min.
- Filter into a 400 ml beaker.
- Wash dish and paper with dry weight and make the volume 100 ml.
- Run a reagent blank in parallel, using 25 ml diluted nitric acid and 75 ml dry weight.
- Add 50 ml quimociac reagent to test beaker, cover with a watch glass, and boil for 1 min (do not use an open flame).
- Cool to room temperature while swirling carefully.
- Transfer the precipitate to the prepared crucible and wash 5 times with 25 ml portions of distilled water.
- Allow each portion to drain thoroughly before adding next portion.

- Dry the crucible and contents at 250°C for 30 min.
- Cool in a dessicator and weigh.

Sample	Weight			Phosphorus (%)
	Sample (W)	Blank (B)	Precipitate (P)	

1.5.1.3 Observations

Calculations

$$\text{Phosphorous (\%)} = \frac{[(P\text{-}B) \times 0.014 \times 1000)]}{W\text{- } (0.0106)\ (\%\ \text{meat protein})}$$

Where,

P = Weight of precipitate (g)

B = Weight of blank (g)

W = Sample weight (g)

0.014 = Gravimetric factor derived from atomic weight of phosphorus = 30.97 divided by the molecular weight of quinolimium phosphomolybdate (QPM) = 2212.71.

0.0106= Factor to correct for the-phosphorus content of meat protein.

1.5.2 Residual phosphates

1.5.2.1 Principle

Total residual phosphorus was estimated in cooked meat samples according to the method of Fiske and Subbarow (1925).

1.5.2.2 Apparatus and chemicals

- Nitric acid, perchloric acid, HCl, Amino naphthol sulphonic acid, sulphuric acid, potassium dihydrogen phosphate.
- Spectrophotometer, conical flask, test tubes etc.

1.5.2.3 Procedure

- Fifty (50) mg of dried cooked meat was digested in corning wide mouth test tube on a burner with 5 ml nitric acid: Perchloric acid (10:1) till all acid got evaporated.
- Added 1ml of cone. HCl and again evaporated, cooled down.
- Added 1% HCl to make volume of 25 mL in the volumetric flask.
- To 2.0 ml of this digested sample, added 2.2 ml distilled water (making the volume to 4.2 ml), 0.2ml of 10N Sulphuric acid, 0.4 ml of 2.5% aqueous solution of Ammonium molybdate and 0.2 ml of Amino-naphthol-sulphonic acid, colour was allowed to develop for 10 min and transmittancy was read at 660 nm in Spectrophotometer.
- The amount of phosphorus in unknown samples calculated on the basis of standard curve by following formula:

$$\text{Conc. of Unkown sample} = \frac{\text{Conc. of Standard} \times \text{O.D. of unknown sample}}{\text{O.D. of known sample}}$$

Calculation

$$\text{Percent Polyphosphate recovered} = \frac{\text{mg Polyphosphate recovered}}{\text{mg Polyphosphate added}} \times 100$$

Standard curve: By using a series of standard phosphorus solutions. For this dissolved 1.099 g Potassium dihydrogen phosphate (KH_2PO_4) in 250mL distilled water which gave standard phosphorus solution containing 1mg phosphorus per ml of solution. One ml of this solution was further diluted to make 100 mL in a volumetric flask with distilled water to give 10µg phosphorus per ml of solution. Standard curve was plotted for 1to10µg phosphorus on the basic of optical density (OD). The colour was developed and measured in the same way as described previously. A blank without any phosphorus was also prepared.

Notes:

- In case of treated samples residual phosphorus was calculated by subtracting total phosphorus of control sample from total FPP.

- Phosphorus of treated samples. Conversion of phosphorus to polyphosphate was done on the basis of mol wt. of polyphosphates.
- For preparation of this solution 0.25g of Aminonaphthol sulphonic acid (ANS) powder was mixed with 97ml of 15% Sodium sulphite solution. After this the remaining ANS was dissolved by adding 20% Sodium sulphite solution (2.5ml). The solution was then filtered through Whatman filter paper No. 1. The solution was kept in dark bottles in refrigerator. It was never used after a week's storage.

2. HPLC method for identification of veterinary drug residues

"Residues" in the widest sense may be defined as undesirable substances present in meat. These substances are chemical or biological in nature and have always been present in a small amount or can be introduced into the environment by various technological practices, can arise as a result of incorrect storage of foodstuff, can get in to the food chain due to modern agricultural practices and thus introduced into the foods or they may be results of medicines given to the animals or of processing methods. Monitoring on the occurrence of residues in meat and their products were relatively a neglected area until last decade. With the advancement of livestock rearing, disease control and intensive crop production system, the chances of residues in foods of animal origin increased tremendously. This results a potential risk of various life threatening diseases such as cancer, leukemia, reproductive disorder besides disruption of body's immune, endocrine and nervous system. Hence, the monitoring residues of emerging toxicants are important to improve national nutritional status by supplying the safe meat foods. Methodology for testing of some important chemical residues/contaminants in meat products are given here.

2.1 Trimethoprim and sulfonamides

Sulfonamides (SAs) are chemotherapeutics most commonly used in veterinary practices, because of their inexpensiveness and wide spectrum antimicrobial activity. Sulfonamides are used in combination with trimethoprim (TMP) in a concentration ratio of 5:1 and these combinations are commonly known as potentiated sulfonamides. SAs act by competing with bacterial p-amino benzoic acid in the enzymatic synthesis of dehydrofolic acid, whereas, trimethoprim, which is a structural analogue of the pteridine dihydrofolic acid is a competitive inhibitor of the enzyme dihydrofolate reductase. This combination of SA and TMP exerts bactericidal effects by decreasing the availability of the reduced foliates that are essential in the synthesis of nucleic acids in the bacteria. However, the presence of residues of TMP and SAs in meat is toxicological and regulatory concern, as some of them could be carcinogenic, cause allergic hypersensitivity reactions and therapeutic ineffectiveness on human beings. Many analytical methods tried for the determination of TMP and SAs in animal tissues. Colorimetric techniques using Bratton-Marshall reagent found to be unsuitable due to lack of sensitivity and selectivity. Other analytical methods based on bioassay, TLC, GC, and HPLC. Greater selectivity and sensitivity could be obtained with TLC methods but have low recovery and poor reproducibility. Although at present many confirmatory LC-MS-MS methods are quoted in the literature, the cost involved in the required instrumentation is high. In comparison to this, HPLC method is simple, rapid, precise, inexpensive, and capable of detecting the residues below MRL (Biswas et al., 2007).

2.2 Apparatus, raw materials and chemicals

- *Meat samples*: Collect about 200 g of composite meat samples, transfer to self-sealing colourless polyethylene bags, label and finally chilled immediately. If not process, store at -20 °C.
- *Chemicals and reagents*. Procure pure standards of trimethoprim (TMP, 99.5%), sulfadimidine (SMZ, 99.7%), sulfadoxine (SDO, 99.8%) and sulfamethoxazole (SMX, 99.8%). Use HPLC grade solvents and chemicals like acetonitrile, ammonium acetate, deionized water etc.
- *Standard stock solutions*: Prepare individual stock solution for each standard. Weigh 10 mg pure standard and dissolve in 1 mL of HPLC grade acetonitrile. Maintain the solutions at 4 °C.
- *Working standard*: Prepare composite working standard solutions of 320, 160, 80, 40, 20, 10, 5, 2.5, 1.25, 0.62 and 0.03µg/mL of each drug in Milli-Q water. Always prepare fresh working standard in each time.
- *Equipments*: HPLC, Milli-Q water purification system, tissue homogenizer, vortex, cooling centrifuge, precolumn/guard

column, reverse phase C_{18} (RP- C_{18}) column, Hamilton syringe etc.

2.3 Procedure

2.3.1 Preparation of sample extract

- Cut the muscle samples (100-150 g) into small pieces after trimmed of external fat and fascia.
- Blend it in a high-speed (15000 rpm) tissue blender for two min.
- Take about 10 g of blended tissue sample into 100 mL polypropylene centrifuge tube.
- Add 10 mL of Milli-Q water and homogenize for 1.5 min using high speed tissue homogenizer.
- Transfer 0.5 g of meat homogenate in a glass test tube, add 1 mL of acetonitrile and then hold the tube for 10 min at room temperature (27±1°C).
- Vortex at high speed for 10 min, centrifuge at 3,500 rpm for 10 min at 4 °C and then collect the supernatant into a separate test tube.
- Re-extract the residues with 1 mL of acetonitrile followed by centrifugation once again as above.
- Filter the supernatant through a 0.22 μm nylon membrane filter and inject 20 μL of the aliquot into the HPLC system.

2.3.2 HPLC-PDA operating conditions

- For the speciation analysis of SA compounds, use a HPLC comprised of a LC-10 AT quaternary gradient pump, Rheodyne manual loop injector with a 20 μL loop, column oven CTO-10AS vp, and a PDA detector.
- Use a reverse phase C_{18} (RP- C_{18}) column (4.6 x 250 mm, i.d.; 5 μm particle size) as stationary phase for separation of TMP, SMZ, SDO and SMX.
- Perform isocratic elution using a mixture of 50 mM ammonium acetate buffer (pH 4.65) -acetonitrile (73:27 v/v) as mobile phase, and monitor the eluent at wavelength of 265 nm with a flow rate of 0.5mL/min at column oven temperature of 40 °C.

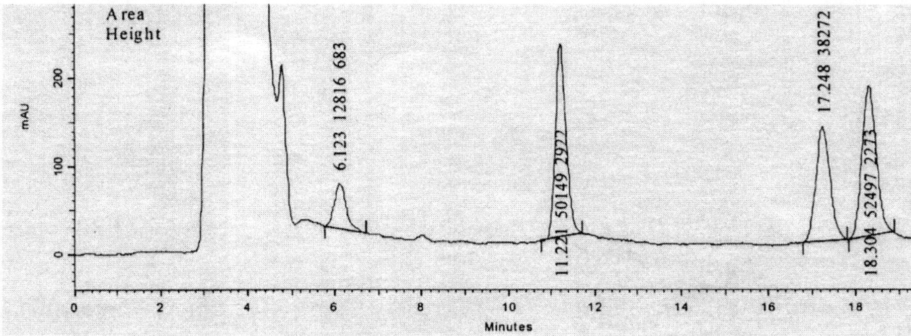

Figure 1. HPLC chromatogram of meat homogenate spiked with 1.0 μg g^{-1} each of, TMP, SMZ, SDO and SMX

- Analyze the data with class-vp 6.12 version software, taking into account the peak heights/areas of analytes.

2.3.3 Preparation of standard calibration curves

- Prepare blank homogenates of meat as described above.
- Prepare a composite working standard solution containing 320 μg/mL each of TMP, SMZ, SDO and SMX from the 1mg/mL of stock solutions and hold at 4°C.
- Make different dilutions with this working standard solution to spike the meat homogenates.
- Spike the blank homogenates of 0.5 g with working standards to obtain final concentrations 2.0, 1.0, 0.5, 0.25, 0.125, 0.062, 0.031 μg/g of TMP, SMZ, SDO and SMX.
- Prepare the sample extract as described previously and inject into HPLC system.
- Prepare a calibration curves after taking measurement of peak height to respective concentrations.
- Use these curves to quantify the residues of TMP, SMZ, SDO and SMX in unknown meat samples by back extrapolation method.

2.3.4 Analytical recovery determination

- Determine analytical recovery by spiking TMP, SMZ, SDO and SMX to blank meat homogenates to yield concentrations of 0.031,

0.25 and 2.0μg/g for TMP; and 0.031, 0.125 and 1.0μg/g for each of SMZ, SDO and SMX.

- Quantify the amount of drug found by the assay method for each concentration using linear regression equation after calibration of standard curves considering peak heights.
- Use at least three determinants for each concentration and then calculate percent recovery.

2.3.5 Precision of the method

- Determine both intra- and inter-day assay precisions by analyzing three spiked concentrations of 0.031, 0.125, 1.0 μg/g, five sets each with blank.
- Determine intra-day assay precision at three occasions at least 6 hrs apart.
- For inter-day assay precision, analyze the samples at least 24 hrs apart for three successive days.
- Use the above standard calibration curves to quantify the residues of TMP, SMZ, SDO and SMX in spiked meat samples by back extrapolation method.

Calculation

Calculate the residues of TMP, SMZ, SDO and SMX by using regression formula after calibration of standard curve.

2.4 Tetracycline, oxytetracycline and chlortetracycline

Antibiotics are used in food producing animals not only to treat disease but also to maintain health and promote growth. Tetracyclines are most widely used antibiotics in veterinary medicine in India due to its broad spectrum of antimicrobial activity, availability and low cost. Unauthorized use of these antibiotics, the failure to follow label directions or inappropriate withdrawal period of time before slaughtering of animals could lead to residues in foods of animal origin, with potential adverse effects on human health. The overuse of OTC/TC/CTC in animal production or their residues in food system poses a potential allergic reaction in sensitized individuals, but sub-therapeutic and therapeutic levels may perturb human gut microflora by introducing resistant strains and altering the metabolic activity of the microflora, its resistant microorganism barrier effects, and its ecological balance without any identified deleterious effects (1-5). Several chromatographic methods have been employed successfully for the monitoring of TCs in tissue samples with different detection modes such as UV-spectrophotometry, fluorescence, and mass spectrometry in the past (6-8). All these procedures used a simple clean-up step by solid phase extraction (SPE) or matrix dispersion. The use of UV detector in residue analysis has low sensitivity, while mass spectrometry still a costly affair. In general, PDA detection is sensitive and has wide scanning range.

2.4.1 Apparatus, raw materials and chemicals

- *Meat samples*: Collect about 200 g of composite meat samples, transfer to self-sealing colourless polyethylene bags, label and finally chilled immediately. If not process, store at -20 °C.
- *Chemicals and reagents*. Pure standard of oxytetracyline (assay 96.2% in HPLC), tetracycline (assay 98.6% in HPLC) and chlortetracycline (assay 97.3% in HPLC) as their hydrochloride, HPLC grade acetonitrile, methanol and water, Nylon filter 0.22 µL filter, AR/GR grade disodium hydrogen phosphate (Na_2HPO_4), citric acid and oxalic acid etc.
- *Standard stock solutions*: Prepare individual stock standard solutions of TCs at 1 mg/mL (free base) in methanol in an amber colour volumetric flask separately and store at -20°C in the dark for maximum period of 2 months.
- *Working standard*: Prepare a composite working standard solution of 320, 160, 80, 40, 20, 10, 5, 2.5, 1.25, 0.625 and 0.031 µg/mL by diluting all stock solutions with methanol. As it is unstable at room temperature, so prepare daily and store at 4°C.
- Mobile phase: Mobile phase for desorption and separation of compounds prepare using a mixture of 0.01 M oxalic acid/ acetonitrile/methanol (77:18:5, v/v/v), and the flow rate was kept at 0.6 mL/min. The detection was performed at 355 nm with scanning range 340-360 nm.
- Prepare 0.01 M oxalic acid (pH 1.6), 0.1 M citric acid and 0.2 M disodium hydrogen phosphate (Na_2HPO_4) buffer in Milli-Q water and filter through 0.22 µm cellulose filter. Prepare 0.01 M

methanolic oxalic acid (pH 1.86) in methanol. Prepare McIlvaine buffer (pH 3.85) by mixing 278 mL of 0.1 M citric acid solution in 222 mL of 0.2 M Na_2HPO_4 solution and adjust the pH to 3.85 with extra citric acid solution. All these buffer solutions were stored at 4°C.

- *Equipments*: HPLC system equipped with a LC-10AT quaternary gradient pump, a Rheodyne manual loop injector 20 µL, a column oven CTO-10AS vp, a PDA detector and a software for data analysis, Milli-Q water purification system, tissue homogenizer, vortex, cooling centrifuge, precolumn/guard column, Analytical column C_8 (RP- C8) column (4.6 × 250 mm, 5 µm particle size), Hamilton syringe etc.

2.4.2 Procedure

2.4.2.1 Preparation of sample extract

- Cut the muscle samples (100-150 g) into small pieces after trimmed of external fat and fascia.
- Blend it in a high-speed (15000 rpm) tissue blender for two min.
- Take about 10 g of blended tissue sample into 100 mL polypropylene centrifuge tube.
- Add 10 mL of Milli-Q water and homogenize for 1.5 min using high speed tissue homogenizer.
- Transfer 0.5 g of meat homogenate in a glass test tube, fortify with 50 µL of variable concentrations of the working standard solution, leaving the analytes in contact with meat sample for 30 min.
- Add 3 mL of McIlvaine buffer, vortex at high speed, incubate for 5 min at room temperature and then centrifuge at 3,500 rpm for 10 min in a refrigerated centrifuge.
- Repeat the extraction by adding 2 mL of McIlvaine buffer and pool the supernatant.
- Filter the supernatant through a 0.22 µm nylon membrane filter and inject 20 µL of the aliquot into the HPLC system.

2.4.2.2 HPLC-PDA operating conditions

- For the speciation analysis of TCs compounds, HPLC system equipped with a LC-10AT quaternary gradient pump, a Rheodyne manual loop injector 20 µL, a column oven CTO-10AS vp, a PDA detector.
- Use a reverse phase C_8 (RP- C_8) column (4.6 x 250 mm, i.d.; 5 µm particle size) as stationary phase for separation of TC, OTC and CTC.
- Perform isocratic elution using a mixture of using a mixture of 0.01 M oxalic acid/acetonitrile/methanol (77:18:5, v/v/v), and the flow rate was kept at 0.6 mL/min. The detection was performed at 355 nm with scanning range 340-360 nm.
- Analyze the data with class-vp 6.12 version software, taking into account the peak heights/areas of analytes.

2.4.2.3 Preparation of standard calibration curves

- Prepare blank homogenates of meat as described above.
- Make different dilutions with this working standard solution to spike the meat homogenates.
- Spike the blank homogenates of 0.5 g with working standards to obtain final concentrations 2.0, 1.0, 0.5, 0.25, 0.125, 0.062, 0.031 µg/g TC, OTC and CTC.
- Prepare the sample extract as described previously and inject into HPLC system.
- Prepare a calibration curves after taking measurement of peak height to respective concentrations.
- Use these curves to quantify the residues of TC, OTC and CTC in unknown meat samples by back extrapolation method.

2.4.2.4 Analytical recovery determination

- Determine analytical recovery by spiking TC, OTC and CTC to blank meat homogenates to yield concentrations of 0.031, 0.25 and 2.0µg/g for each of TC, OTC and CTC.

- Quantify the amount of drug found by the assay method for each concentration using linear regression equation after calibration of standard curves considering peak heights.
- Use at least three determinants for each concentration and then calculate percent recovery.

2.4.2.5 Precision of the method

- Determine both intra- and inter-day assay precisions by analyzing three spiked concentrations of 0.031, 0.125, 1.0 μg/g, five sets each with blank.
- Determine intra-day assay precision at three occasions at least 6 hrs apart.

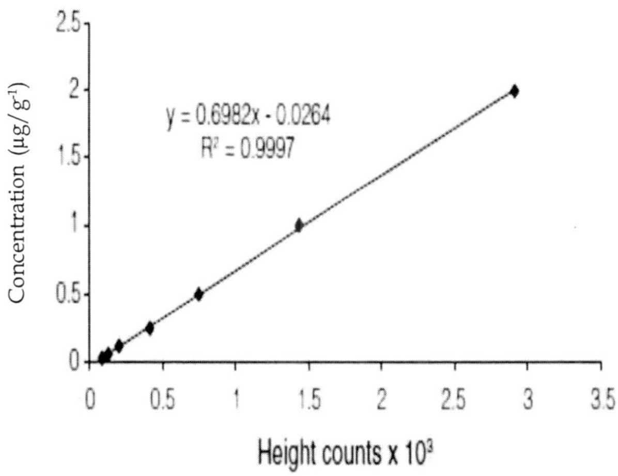

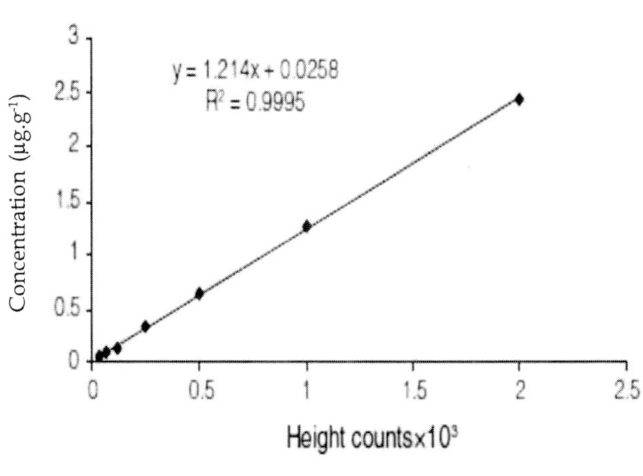

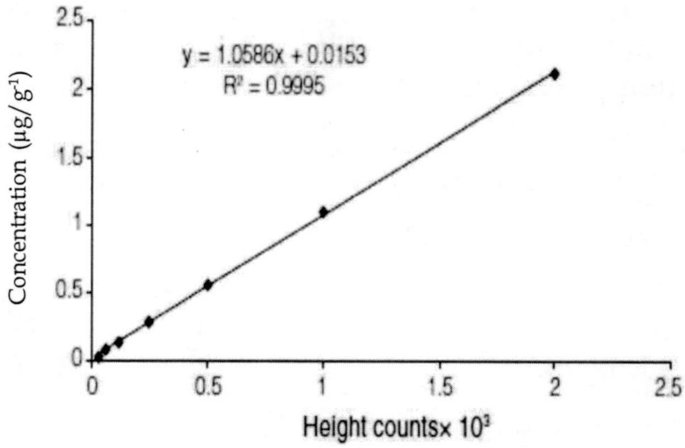

Figure 2. Linear calibration curve of the HPLC method for oxytetracycline, tetracycline, and chlortetracycline residues in meat.

- For inter-day assay precision, analyze the samples at least 24 hrs apart for three successive days.
- Use the above standard calibration curves to quantify the residues of TC, OTC and CTC in spiked meat samples by back extrapolation method.

3. HPLC method for identification of pesticide residues

3.1 Carbaryl

Carbaryl insecticide is one of the extensively used chemicals in agricultural field for crop protection, as ectoparasiticidal, and regular household practices. This is because of their high and broad insecticidal efficacy but low toxicity towards variety of warm-blooded animals. This compound is less persistent than organochlorine pesticides and produces fewer or no toxicological products. However, the presence of residues of carbaryl in meat is of toxicological and regulatory concern as it could be acetylcholinesterase inhibitor and cause allergic hypersensitivity reactions in human beings. Therefore, both legislators and consumers have shown increased interest in the safety of food products. As the established tolerance for carbaryl insecticide in meat is low (100 ppb) and metabolism in animals is high (JECFA, 2002), many analytical method is developed for monitoring of carbaryl residues in meat. Methods for analysis of carbaryl insecticide are tried by using gas chromatography (GC), liquid chromatography (LC) with flurogenic labeling technique (Page and French, 1992), LC with reverse-phase separation followed by a post column derivatization (Nunes et al., 1998) and HPLC techniques (Biswas et al., 2010). Post column derivatization with fluorescence detection in LC and liquid chromatography-mass spectrometry (LC-MS) has high sensitivity and selectivity, but methods are complicated, expensive, and also required exhaustive cleanup techniques (Ozhan et al., 2003; Bogialli et al., 2004). The method describes by Biswas et al. (2010) is relatively simple, inexpensive and required only little toxic solvents and involved simple sample extraction and cleanup steps. The sample deproteinized with acetonitrile, cleanup on aminopropyl-bonded silica cartridge and determined by photo-diode-array (PDA) detector. The method also partially validated for detection of carbaryl residue in meat samples.

3.1.1 Apparatus, chemicals and reagents

- HPLC equipped with PDA detector
- Milli-Q water purification system
- Guard column
- Centrifuge machine
- Votex machine
- Tissue homogenizer
- Filtration unit with nitrocellulose filter (0.45 μm)
- Pure standard of carbaryl (1-napthyl methyl carbamate; assay 99.7%)
- HPLC grade acetonitrile
- Methanol
- HPLC grade water (Deionized water)
- Standard stock solution: Dissolve at 1mg of carbaryl standard in 1 mL prepared by HPLC grade water and solution was maintained at 4°C in the dark
- Working standard solution: Prepare working standard in mobile phase [a mixture of acetonitrile-water (50:50, v/v)]. Working standard at concentrations of 320, 160, 80, 40, 20, 10, 5, 2.5, 1.25, 0.62 and 0.3μg/mL carbaryl prepare fresh and stored at 4^0C.

3.1.2 Procedure

3.1.2.1 Preparation of sample extract

- Collect carbaryl free muscle sample from the animals slaughtered as per standard method.
- Remove excessive connective tissues, fascia etc from the samples and cut in to fine pieces.
- Blend the samples in a high speed (15,000 rpm) tissue blender for 2 min.
- Weigh ten grams of blended sample, transfer into a 100 mL polypropylene centrifuge tube.
- Add 10 mL of Milli-Q water, mix well and then homogenize for 1.5 min using a high speed tissue homogenizer.
- Weigh accurately 0.5 g of meat homogenate in a glass test tube by dispensing homogenate with the help of micropipette of 5000 μL capacity.
- Prepare a total 10 test tubes of meat homogenate.
- Spike 50 μL of the working standard to meat homogenate in each test tube with the increasing concentration.
- The final concentrations of carbary in decreasing order will be 8.0, 4.0, 2.0, 1.0, 0.5, 0.25, 0.125, 0.062, 0.031 and 0.015μg/g.
- Add 1.5 mL of acetonitrile hold for 15 min at room temperature (27 ± 1°C), vortex for 1.5 min and then keep mixture 5 min undisturbed.
- Add 1 mL of water, vortex again at high speed for 1 min and thereafter centrifuge at 3,000 rpm for 15 min in a refrigerated centrifuge.
- Collect supernatant into a separate test tube.
- Filter the aliquot by using 0.22μm nylon filter and store at 4±1°C.

3.1.2.2 HPLC condition

- For the analysis of carbaryl, a high-performance liquid chromatograph composed of an LC-10 AT quaternary gradient pump, a Rheodyne manual loop injector with a 20 μL loop, a column oven CTO-10AS vp, and a PDA detector.

- Use a reverse phase C_{18} (RP-C_{18}) stainless steel column (250 × 4.6 mm i.d), 5 µm particle size, 100 A^0 pore size with matching guard column as stationary phase.
- Run the mobile phase- a mixture of acetonitrile-water (50:50; v/v) for conditioning the column and setting the base line.
- Monitor the eluent at a wavelength of 220 nm with a flow rate of 0.9 mL/min at a column oven temperature of 35°C.

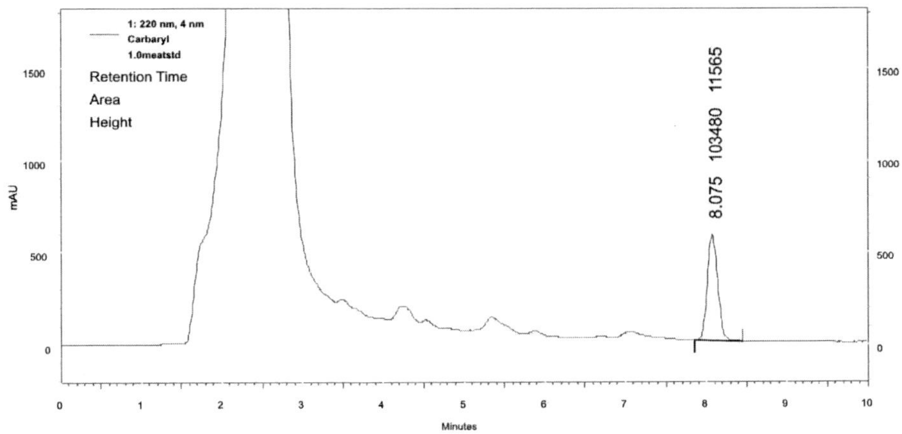

Figure 3. Liquid chromatogram of carbaryl spiked (1.0 µg/g) meat homogenates

- Inject 50 mL of aliquot into the LC column equipped with pre-column/guard column.
- Wait to complete the run.
- Analyze the data with class-vp 6.12 version software, taking into account the peak heights/peak areas of analyte.

3.1.2.3 Recovery, precision, LOD and LOQ determination

- Determine analytical recovery by calculating concentration found vs concentration spiked. Perform at least five determinants for each concentration (high, medium and low) to determine the percent recovery
- Determine analytical precision of the method by evaluating intra- and inter day assay precisions at three spiked concentrations of 0.02, 0.1, and 0.5µg/g, five sets each with blank.

- Determine intraday assay precision at three occasions at least 6 h apart
- Determine inter-day ass precision at least 24 h apart for three successive days.
- Calculate limits of detection (LOD) as the amount corresponding to mean value plus three times the standard deviation for the blank sample i.e. with a signal to noise-ration of 3 (S/N-3).

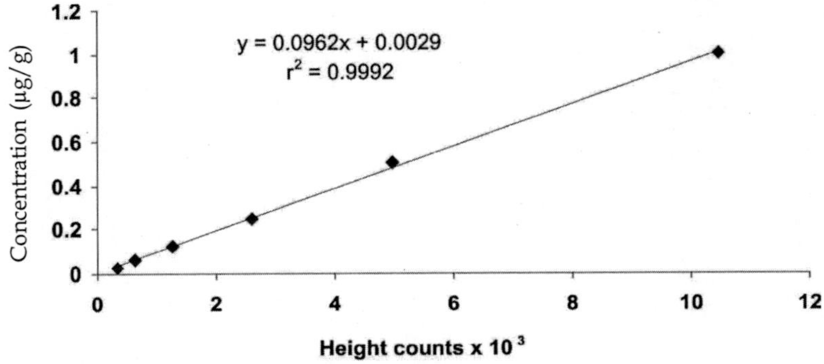

Figure 4. Standard calibration curve for carbaryl residues

- Measure the limits of quantification (LOQ) from where standard calibration curve was satisfied. Calculate the LOQ from the minimal accepted value of the signal to noise ratio of 6 (S/N 6).

Calculation

- Prepare a standard calibration curve ($y = 0.0962x + 0.0029$, $r^2 = 0.9992$) by taking peak height to the respective concentrations.
- Use the formula to quantify the residues of carbaryl in the meat samples analyzed.

3.2 Cypermethrin and deltamethrin

Synthetic pyrethroids are extensively used chemicals in agricultural field for crop protection, as ectoparasiticidal, and regular household practices. The reason for this is that they prove to have high and broad insecticide efficacy but low toxicity towards variety of warm-blooded animals. In addition, this compound is less persistent than organochlorine pesticides and produces fewer toxic degradation products. However, cypermethrin and deltamethrin insecticides are acetylcholinesterase inhibitor, so they are considered to be toxic for human beings. Various chromatographic methods employed to determine cypermethrin, deltamethrin and other pyrethroids in corn, food including meat, and environmental sample (Chen and Wang, 1996). A simple HPLC with radiometric (HPLC-RAM) detection techniques was also explained for determination of tralomethrin, deltamethrin and decamethrinic acid (Br_2CH) in fish tissue (Mao et al., 1993). The separation of these compounds was achieved using hexane/dioxane gradient solvent system on a normal-phase silica column. Similarly, other researchers also analysed animal tissue samples by using HPLC system (Pavan et al., 1999, Anderson, 1983 and Stephenson, 1982). But all these procedure adopted previously are time consuming, requires exhaustive extraction and clean up, cost effective and also pertained complexities in the instrumentation. A simple method developed by Biswas et al. (2009) to better quantification of these compounds using HPLC method as under-

3.2.1 Apparatus, raw materials and chemicals

- *Meat samples*: Collect about 200 g of composite meat samples, transfer to self-sealing colourless polyethylene bags, label and finally chilled immediately. If not process, store at -20 °C.
- *Reagents, solvents and standards*: Pure standard of cypermethrin (mixture of isomers; assay 96.7%) and deltamethrin (assay 99.9%), HPLC grade acetonitrile, methanol and water, nitrocellulose filter 0.22 μm.
- *Standard stock solutions*: Prepare cypermethrin and deltamethrin free base concentration (1 mg/mL) in HPLC grade acetonitrile, separately.
- *Working standard*: Prepare separate working standard solutions of 12, 6, 3, 1.5, 0.75, 0.38, and 0.19 μg/mL each of cypermethrin and deltamethrin in mobile phase daily.
- *Mobile phase*: Use isocratic elution of a mixture of acetonitrile and Milli-Q water in the proportion of 60: 40 (v/v).
- *LC system*: Use LC system comprised of Varian 6.12 Class-vp software, LC-10 AT quaternary gradient pump, Rheodyne manual loop injector with a 20 μL loop, column oven CTO-10 AS vp and photo-diode-array (PDA) detector. Take absorbance at 220 nm.

- *Column*: RP-C18 (250×4.6 mm id) stainless steel column, 4 μm particle size, 100 angstrom pore size, with matching guard column supplied with column.
- *Apparatus*: HPLC equipped with PDA detector, Milli-Q water purification system, Centrifuge machine, Votex machine , Tissue homogenizer, Filtration unit with nitrocellulose filter (0.22μm) etc.

3.2.2 Procedure

3.2.2.1 Preparation of sample extract

- Collect carbaryl free muscle sample from the animals slaughtered as per standard method.
- Remove excessive connective tissues, fascia etc from the samples and cut in to fine pieces.
- Blend the samples in a high speed (15,000 rpm) tissue blender for 2 min.
- Weigh ten grams of blended sample, transfer into a 100 mL polypropylene centrifuge tube.
- Add 10 mL of Milli-Q water, mix well and then homogenize for 1.5 min using a high speed tissue homogenizer.
- Weigh accurately 0.5 g of meat homogenate in a glass test tube by dispensing homogenate with the help of micropipette of 5000 μL capacity.
- Prepare a total 10 test tubes of meat homogenate.
- Spike 50 μL of cypermethrin and deltamethrin, working standard solution (25 μL each).
- Allow to stand the tubes at room temperature for 20 min.
- Add 2 mL of acetonitrile, vortex-mixing at high speed for 1.5 min, hold the tubes again at room temperature for 10 min, and finally centrifuge at 3,000 rpm for 20 min in a refrigerated centrifuge.
- Transfer the clear supernatant to separate graduated test tubes and add half the volume of HPLC grade water and vortex again for 1 min.
- Centrifuge the tubes at 10,000 rpm for 10 min.

- Collect the supernatant in micro centrifuge tubes and inject into the column.

3.2.2.2 HPLC condition

- Perform separation of cypermethrin and deltamethrin using a reverse phase C_{18} (RP-C_{18}) column as stationary phase and a mixture of HPLC water-acetonitrile (40:60, v/v) as mobile phase.
- Adjust the flow rate of mobile phase at 0.6 mL/min with the column oven temperature of 40°C.
- Monitor both the eluents at wavelength of 220 nm.

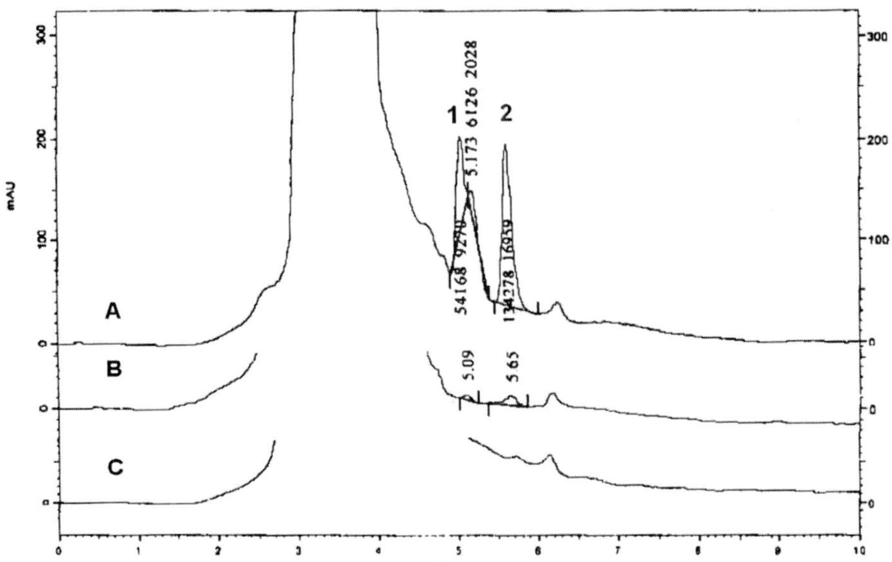

Figure 5. Chromatogram of cypermethrin and deltamethrin

- Run the HPLC for at least 30 min to adjust the base-line of the chromatogram.
- Inject 50 mL of aliquot into the LC column equipped with pre-column/guard column.
- Wait to complete the run.
- Analyze the data with available software with the HPLC system, taking into account the peak heights/peak areas of analyte.

3.2.2.3 Recovery, precision, LOD and LOQ determination

- Determine analytical recovery of cypermethrin and deltamethrin by calculating concentration found vs concentration spiked. Perform recovery study at least five determinants at three fortification levels (0.02, 0.15, 1.2 ppm) to determine the percent recovery.
- For intra-day assay precision (repeatability), fortify/spiking the working standard at 0.04, 0.08, 0.15 ppm concentrations five sets each with blank. Analyze the extract at three occasions at least 6 h apart.
- Inter-day assay precision (reproducibility) determines at spiking levels of 0.04, 0.15 and 1.2 ppm of meat samples, five sets each with blank. Determine inter-day assay precision at least 24 h apart for three successive days.
- Calculate limits of detection (LOD) as the amount corresponding to mean value plus three times the standard deviation for the blank sample i.e. with a signal to noise-ration of 3 (S/N-3).
- Measure the limits of quantification (LOQ) from where standard calibration curve was satisfied. Calculate the LOQ from the minimal accepted value of the signal to noise ratio of 6 (S/N 6).

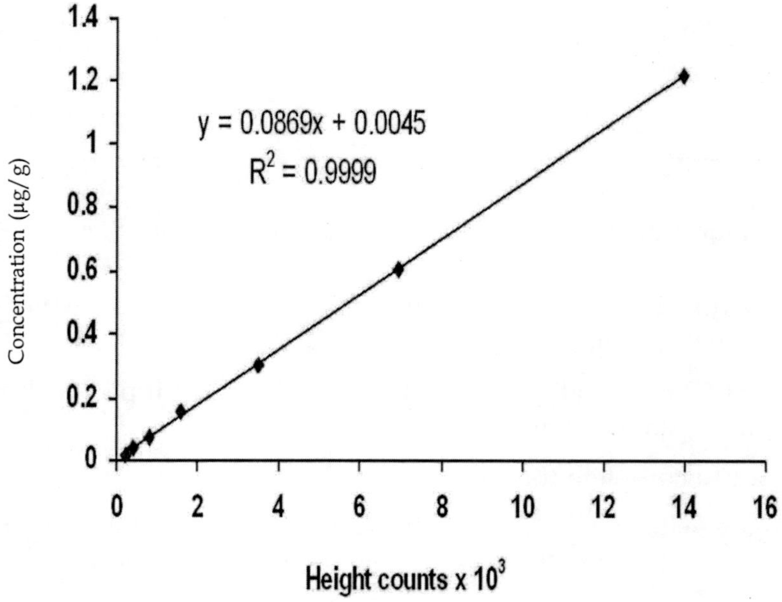

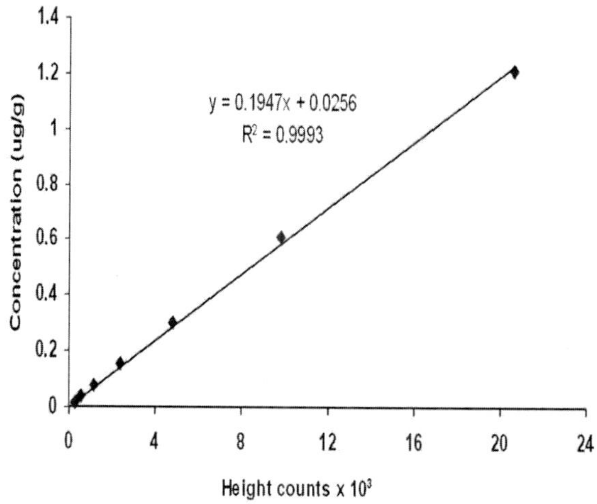

Figure 6. Standard calibration curve for determination of cypermethrin and deltamethrin

Calculation

- Prepare standard calibration curves (y = 0.0869x + 0.0045; r^2 = 0.9999 for cypermethrin, and y = 0.1947x + 0.0256; r^2 = 0.9993 for deltamethrin; y = peak height, x=cypermethrin/deltamethrin concentration, and r^2 = correlation coefficient) spiking a mixture of cypermethrin and deltamethrin compounds in tissue homogenates at 0.02, 0.04, 0.08, 0.16, 0.32, 0.64 and 1.2 ppm concentration.
- Calculate the concentration considering peak height of peak area of respective compounds for each sample.

References

Biswas, A. K., Rao, G. S., Kondaiah, N., Anjaneyulu, A. S. R. and Malik, J. K. (2007). *J Agric and Food Chem* 55(22): 8845-8850.

Biswas, A. K., Kondaiah, N., Anjaneyulu, A. S. R. and Rao, G.S. (2009). *Fleischwirtschaft- International* 24(1): 82-86.

Biswas, A. K., Kondaiah, N., Anjaneyulu, A. S. R., Rao, G. S. and Singh, R. P. (2010). *Analytical Methods* 2: 393-396.

Andrade, R., Reyes, F. G. R. and Rath, S. (2005). *Food Chem* 91: 173–179

Fiske, C.H and Sabbarow, Y 1925. *J. Biol. Chem.* 66: 375

❑❑❑

Chapter IX

Rapid Test for Identification of Meat Quality

1. Physical examination of meat

- The visual physical inspection is done for any change in appearance and colour, flavour or odour, physical damage etc.
- **Appearance & colour:** In general, colour of meat is influenced by variation in species and state of Fe ion in myoglobin pigment of muscles; the raw fresh meat is bright red in colour whereas cured meat has typical pink colour. Any change in colour may occur accidentally during dressing (Bile pigments), absorbed colour or paint from packaging, erosion colour or due to microbial contamination. Various fungi or bacteria such *as Pseudomonas, Candida, Aspergillums, and Rhizopus* etc lead to changes in colour of meat.
- **Flavour or odour:** The changes in typical meat flavour may occur due to putrefactive changes or absorbed odour from foreign material. Any change in odour is a clear indication of spoilage of meat.
- **Physical state:** The slime formation or whiskers occur due to microbial contaminations, which indicate the spoilage of meat and meat products.

2. Test for inefficiency of bleeding (Malachite green test)

2.1 Principle

- The test is based on the principle that oxidized haemoglobin on addition of acid solution of malachite green produces a green colour complex. This test can be used to know the bleedi efficacy and also to identify meat from cold slaughtered animal (dead animal), from that of meat obtained from healthy live animal. In the case of cold slaughtered meat there is high blood content in the subcutaneous blood vessels, the amount of oxidized haemoglobin content is more which forms a green coloured complex with acid malachite green.

2.2 Requirements

- 0.1 % aqueous malachite green solution (pH 5.3).
- Meat extract (meat: distilled water, 1:2 ratio) or meat sample.

2.3 Procedure

- Take 1 -2 g of meat sample or 1- 2 mL meat extract.
- Add 0.4 mL malachite green solution.
- Mix properly and observe for green colour development.
- Development of intense dark green colour indicates less bleeding efficiency.

3. Resazurin test (Dye reduction test)

3.1 Background

- This test estimates bacterial population in meat sample indirectly. Microbes enzymes are capable of reduction reaction. Resazurin dye is commonly used as indicator dye because it has high pictorial value and imparts characteristic blue colour. It is based on the principle of reduction of resazurin indicated by change in colour from dark blue to purple and finally faded pink colour.

3.2 Requirements

- Sterilized graduated test tubes, Homogenizer/blender/pestle & mortar, Sterilized pipettes, Clock, Water bath.
- Sterilized standard resazurin solution: prepare 0.05 per cent (w/v) stock solution by dissolving resazurin in glass distilled water and store under refrigerator in amber coloured bottle. Prepare 0.005 per cent working solution by diluting stock solution with distilled water and use within 6 hours.

3.3 Procedure

- Take 10 g raw meat sample free from bones, fascia etc.
- Add 50ml sterilized distilled water.
- Homogenize it in sterile pestle and mortar.
- Take 10ml of homogenate in graduated test tubes under aseptic conditions.
- Add 1ml of working solution of resazurin (0.005%) to homogenate.
- Close the test tube with sterilized glass stopper and mix the content thoroughly.
- Incubate the test tube in a water bath maintained at 37°C.
- Run a blank i.e. without dye along with the sample throughout the experiment.
- Remove the test tubes after 1 hour.
- Check the change in colour and then again keep the test tube in hot water bath and check again after every half hour interval and compare it with blank.
- Interpret the results.

Reduction Time	**Meat Quality**
10 minutes	Not acceptable
10-30 minutes	May be acceptable
30-60 minutes	Good quality
Over 60 minutes	Very good quality

Notes:

- Use sterilized glassware for the tests.
- Transfer the sample and dye under aseptic conditions in test tube near flame of Bunsen burner.
- Do not expose stock solution of resazurin and test tubes to direct sunlight.

4. Rimington and fowrie test (Jaundice test)

- Take 2 g of fat in a test tube.
- Add 5 mL of 5 % NaOH solution and boiled it for one min, shake frequently and cool under tap water.
- Add equal volume of ether and allow to settle.
- In positive case, water soluble sodium salt formed (green colour) during reaction will be deposited at the bottom. If physiological yellow colour of fat is present the upper layer is yellow, while with both billirubin and other pigment (carotene) an upper yellow and bottom yellowish green layers are formed.

5. Nitrazine-yellow test

- The test determines the acidity of meat. For this, take a piece of meat free of blood, fat and connective tissue in a Petri dish and nitrazine yellow indicator (1:10000) sufficient to cover the meat. Mix with a stirring rod. Note the colour change with standard chart provided.

pH	Colour	Inference
6.0	Yellow	Good Keeping quality
6.4	Olive green	Not having same good quality
6.8	Bluish violet	Suspect of signs of incipient spoilage.

6. Water protein ratio

- Water protein ratio in muscle is generally constant and not affected by the fat content. In extremely emaciated animals, the percentage of water present in the muscle is about 80 percent and protein 19 percent giving a water protein ration of 4:1, in lean meat water is 76.5 per cent and protein about 22 percent, and the water protein ration is less than 4:1. This test is very useful to differentiate between lean and emaciated animals.

7. Test for abnormal odour

7.1 Boiling test

- A pan is filled with cold water and a piece of meat about the size of palm of the hand is put on it. Lid is replaced and is put on the flame for boiling.
- When boiling starts, the lid is removed and odour is smelled. If abnormal odour is present the meat also has abnormal taste and if necessary the meat and water should be tested.

7.2 Frying test

- The test is suitable for determining the suitability of fatty tissues for marketing. When testing lean meats, a small amount of clean fat may be added previously to the frying pan. Rancid fat will give off odour on frying.

8. Copper sulphate test

- The test is done to detect the staleness of meat. For detection, take 10 g finely ground meat and add 30 mL of distilled water boil and filter through cotton. Cool to room temperature and take 5 mL of the filtrate and add 4 drops of 1 % $CuSO_4$ solution.
  - Clear broth indicates fresh meat.
  - Turbid broth indicates doubtful.
  - Deep turbid broth indicates stale of unfit or consumption.

9. Meat swelling capacity

- This test determines the freshness of meat. Swelling capacity of meat increases during spoilage due to protein degradation and penetration of more amounts of water in protein matrix. Blend 25 g of meat with 100 mL of distilled water for 2 min. Centrifuge 35 mL of homogenate at 2000 rpm for 15 min. Measure the amount of supernatant (S) and pellet.

Calculation

% Meat swelling capacity = $(35\text{-}S\text{-}7)/7\times100$.

10. Differentiation of chilled and thawed frozen meat

10.1 Background

- This test is used to differentiate chilled and frozen thawed frozen meat as some suppliers sell thawed frozen meat as chilled meat, since the former is likely to be poor keeping quality and liable to spoilage and rancidity, it is important that the two be differentiated.
- Two tests are available such as photometric and colour test. Both of which are measure the concentration of a mitochondrial enzyme (β–hydroxyacyl CoA – dehydrogenase – HADH) in meat juice. The HADH activity is higher in frozen meat because freezing ruptures mitochondria, which releases this enzyme into meat juice.

Species	Photometric method		Colour test	
	Dilution of meat press juice	*HADH activity U/mL in frozen meat*	*Dilution of meat press juice*	*Reaction time in minute*
Beef	1:200	>3.5	1:100	60
Veal	1:200	>3.5	1:100	60
Pork	1:200	>6.0	1:100	30
Mutton	1:200	>5.0	1:100	45
Chicken (breast meat)	1:200	>5.0	1:100	60
Duck (breast meat)	1:400	>20.0	1:400	40
Goose (breast meat)	1:400	>20.0	1:400	40
Turkey (breast meat)	1:200	>5.0	1:100	60

10.2 Preparation of meat press juice

- Take 10 g of intact thawed meat sample and place it in between two glass or plastic Petri plates. Give equal and adequate pressure from either side of both the Petri plates so that meat juice comes out. Collect the meat press juice and store at – 18 °C, if not analyzed immediately.

10.2.1 Method I (Photometric method)

10.2.1.1 Requirements

- 0. 1 M phosphate buffer (pH 6.0)
- 34.4 mM EDTA
- 7. 5 mM β–nicotinamide adenine dinucleotide reduced form (β-NADH) grade III
- 5.9 mM acetoacetyl – CoA – enzyme A.

10.1.1.2 Procedure

- Take 0.1 mL diluted meat juice (1:200).
- Add 2.6 mL of 0.1 M phosphate buffer, 0.2 mL 34.4 mM EDTA and 0.05 mL of 7.5 mM β-NADH.
- Start the reaction by adding 0.05 mL of 5.9 mM acetoacetyl CoA enzyme.
- Mix and immediately read extinction at 340 nm wavelength against air.
- Wait for 3 min and take reading of extinction at 340 nm at 25 °C.
- Calculate the decrease in extinction per min (DE/min)
- Express HADH activity as IU per mL press juice.

Calculation

U/mL= V/E × D × n

Where, V= volume of the text mixture

E= extinction coefficient for NADH at 340 nm (6.3)

D= light path of cuvette (1 cm)

n= volume of meat juice (0.1 mL)

U/mL=3/6.3 × 1 × 0.1 × (DE/min) × 200.

10.2.2 Method II (colour test)

10.2.2.1 Requirements

- 0. 1 M phosphate buffer (pH 6.0)

- 34.4 mM EDTA
- 1. 5 mM β–nicotinamide adenine dinucleotide reduced form (β-NADH) grade III.
- 0.28 % Meldolablue solution.
- 5.9 mM acetoacetyl – CoA – enzyme A.

10.2.2.2 Procedure

- Take 0.1 mL diluted meat juice (1:100) in a test tube.
- Add 2.4 mL of 0.1 M phosphate buffer, 0.2 mL 34.4 mM EDTA, 0.2 mL of 1.5 mM β-NADH, 0.12 mL of 5.9 mM acetoacetyl CoA enzyme.
- Mix properly and leave the tube in the dark for 1 h.
- Add 0.1 mL meldolablue solution and shake for 30 sec.
- If the solution remains colourless the meat is fresh and meat it turns purple the meat is frozen thawed.
- After 45 sec fresh sample will go purple due to oxidation of meldolablue by air.

❑❑❑

Chapter X

Methods for Species Differentiation of Meat

Authenticity testing of meat products is important for labelling and assessment of value and is therefore necessary to avoid unfair competition and assure consumers protection against fraudulent practices commonly observed in the food industry. In the case of meat, it has been reported that meat from some species fetched low commercial values than their corresponding related species, and again meat from female of same species has little demand by the consumers due to their poor eating quality and aesthetic values. Some malscrupolous meat processors are adulterating costlier meat with meat from closely related low-cost species or even meat from female animals mixing with male. This falsification or adulteration of meat is misleading the people to lose their faith on packaged food items. The accurate labelling of meat products is mandated and monitored by Bureau of Indian Standard (BIS) and Food safety and Standard Authority of India under Food Safty and Standards Act 2006.

The consumption of undeclared meat may lead to immunological reaction (allergic) to the sensitized individuals; hurt the religious sentiments of various communities who are prejudiced of different kinds of meat, also leads to havoc economic loss to the meat industry. However, adulterations refer not only to the replacement of meat ingredients but also to inappropriate information concerning the origin of other raw materials. These include replacement of ingredients in a product, most frequently, by cheaper meat species; addition of undeclared constituents of animal origin, proportion of ingredients incompatible with the product label or specification; sale of fresh meat that had earlier been frozen; improper labelling of the geographic origin of the products.

As per an estimate about 25-30% of meat sold in India is adulterated. So it is necessary to authenticate meat adopting simple, sensitive, low cost and reliable analytical techniques for consumer safety. Researchers tried to establish a fruitful tool for identification of adulterated meat, however, a challenging task for the food inspectors. Presence of meat in any sample can be easily established on the basis of 3-methyl histidine content of muscle. This amino acid however, is common to all meats and thus cannot be used as a marker for species recognization. The rapid tests for meat species identification under field conditions have been developed by various workers in past. Some of techniques are given as followings-

Methods/techniques

- Various methods have been developed for identification of species origin of meat and meat products. These include-
  - Physical techniques
  - Anatomical techniques
  - Histological techniques
  - Chemical techniques
  - Biological or serological or immunological techniques
  - ELISA
  - Electrophoresis techniques
  - Molecular techniques

1. Physical techniques

- *General appearance:* Colour, consistency, odour.
- *General characteristics of the body fat:* Colour, consistency, quality etc.

Table 1. Quality characteristics of meat of different animals

Meat	General appearance			
	Colour	Consistency	Odour	Marbling
Beef	Dark red with slight brownish tinge	Firm and cut surface are shiny	-	Present
Buffalo meat	Dark red	Firm	-	Absent or poorly present
Veal	Pale grey to greyish red	Firm	-	Absent
Chevon	Light red and paler than mutton	Very firm	Goaty odour	Absent
Mutton	Dark red	Firm and dense	Ammonical	Absent to scanty
Pork	Grayish white to light red	Very soft	Urine like	Present
Poultry meat	White	Firm	-	Absent
Horse meat	Dark red with bluish tinge	Firm with prominent fascia	-	Absent
Camel meat	Red	Fairly firm	-	Absent
Dog meat	Dark meat	Firm	Disagreeable and repulsive	Slightly present
Rabbit meat	Pale, grey to grey red	Firm	Pronounced	Absent
Venison	Dark red to brownish red	-	-	Absent or very less

Table 2. Quality characteristics of fat of different animal species

Fat	Colour	Consistency	Fat type	Remark
Beef	Yellowish white	Firm	Intramuscular fat	-
Buffalo fat	Pure white	Slightly firm	No intramuscular fat	-
Veal	Reddish yellow to white	Loose and grey	No intramuscular fat	-
Chevon	Pure white	Hard , firm and brittle	No intramuscular fat	-
Mutton	Pure white	Hard, firm and brittle	Abundant intermuscular fat	-
Pork	White	Soft and greasy	Subcutaneous but intramuscular also	On boiling it turns to whitish grey
Poultry fat	Yellow	Loose	Mostly subcutaneous	-
Horse fat	In young –light gold to yellow In mature -white	Soft and greasy	No intramuscular fat	On exposure to a ir turns to blackish
Dog fat	White to whitish grey	Oily and greasy	Slight intramuscular	-
Rabbit fat	Whitish yellow	Loose	Fat is absent in muscle and confined to body cavity	-

Table 3. Differentiation of beef and buffalo meat based on physicochemical characteristics

Characteristics	Beef	Buffalo meat
Colour	Dark red with slight brownish tinge	Dark red
Meat consistency	Firm and cut surface are shiny	Firm
Marbling	Present	Absent or poorly present
Fat colour	Yellowish white	Pure white
Fat consistency	Firm	Slightly firm
Location of fat	Intramuscular	Mostly inter-muscular
Carotene content	Present	Absent

2. Anatomical techniques

- This technique is applicable only when carcasses are intact conditions as osseous structure give some indication of speciation. Deboned or minced meat can be differentiated by using this technique. The primary identification method for meat species is
  - Dental formula if teeth are attached with the carcass.
  - Bone percentage of carcasses
  - Rib numbers and their degree of curvature
  - Characteristics of long bones
- To identify the meat of male and female animals of different species, the presence of gonads, udder and developed gracilis confirm meat from female gender while carcass containing bulbocavernosus muscle indicate meat from male animals. The size of pelvic cavity in female animal's carcasses will be larger than male animals.

2.1 Dentition

S.No	Species		Permanent dentition	
1	Cattle and buffalo	(0033)	2– – –=32	(4033)
2	Sheep and goat	(0033)	2– – –=32	(4033)
3	Pig	(3143)	2– – –=44	(3143)
4	Horse	(3133)	2– – –=40	(3133)

2.2 Bone percentage of carcass

Proportion of bones in dressed carcasses can give indication of animal species

S.No.	Species	Percentage of bone
1	Mutton	25
2	Bobby calves	50
3	Veal calves	25
4	Pork	12-20
5	Bull	15

2.3 Ribs on thorax

Paired ribs vary in number in different species of animals

S.No.	Species	Ribs in pairs	Sternal ribs
1	Ox	13	8
2	Pig	14-15	7
3	Sheep and goat	13	8
4	Horse	18	8
5	Dog	13	9

2.4 Characteristics of long bones

Bone	Species	Characteristics
Scapula	Sheep	Short and broad, superior spine thickness and bent back.
	Goat	Possesses distinct neck spine, straight and narrow.
Radius	Sheep	1.25 times length of metacarpus.
	Goat	Twice the length of metacarpus.
Ulna	Horse	Extends only 1/2th length of radius.
	Ox	Extends and articulates with carpus.
Femur	Horse	There is no third trochanter. Fibula is only a small point projection.
	Ox	Possesses third trochanter. Fibula extends 2/3rd the length of tibia.

3. Histological techniques

- These techniques generally measure
  - Muscle fibre length.
  - Muscle fibre diameter.
  - Density and pattern of the muscle fibres.
- The procedure for determination of muscle fibre diameter is given preceding chapter can also lead to species identification. Following characteristics should consider for species differentiation of beef and buffalo meat. Same also consider for other closely related species too.

Characteristics	**Beef**	**Buffalo meat**
Muscle fibre diameter	Larger	Smaller
Number of muscle fibres per mm^3	Less	More
Muscle striation	Less angular	More angular

4. Chemical techniques

- For meat speciation various chemical tests have of immense value. These tests estimate the amount of certain chemicals presents in the meat of different animal species. These methods obviate difficulties arises for anatomical method of speciation but have not yet get popularity due to component of meat undergoes different biochemical or physical changes after heating.
  - *Composition of meat*: Measure intramuscular fat of different species since it varies according to the meat species. The intramuscular fat in mutton is higher (13.3 per cent) as compared to beef (2.6 per cent), buffalo meat (0.9 per cent), chevon (3.6 per cent) and pork (4.4 per cent). Vitamin A is present in beef and mutton absent in buffalo meat, chevon or pork.
  - *Myoglobin content*: Determine myoglobin content as per methodology as given in the chapter. Horse flesh contains maximum myoglobin content (0.71 per cent), much higher than the musculature of other animals.

- *Glycogen content*: Measure the glycogen content as per procedure given in the Chapter IV(7). Horse flesh is richer in glycogen as compared to most food animals.
- *Composition of body fats:*

a) Refractive index: Horse fat has higher refractive index (53.5) than ox (less than 40) and pig (less than 50) fat.

b) Iodine number: Iodine number of horse fat (70-85) is higher than even lard (50–70), whereas, iodine number of ox and sheep fat is 35-46.

c) Carotene content: Estimate the carotene content following method as given in chapter VI(3.1). Buffalo fat is white due to Absence of carotene whereas cow fat is cream to yellow in colour due to carotene content.

d) Fatty acid analysis: Determine fatty acid composition by GLC method as given in Chapter II(3.5). Horse fat contains 1-2 per cent linoleic acid, whereas, other fats contain less than 0.1 per cent linoleic acid.

5. Molecular techniques (PCR based techniques)

Analysis of DNA rather than protein has been exploited for species identification due to its stability at high temperature and have conversed structure within all tissues of individual. In animal cell, DNA present in nucleus and mitochondria. The mitochondrial DNA is more conversed in different species of animals. Cytochrome b gene is most commonly targeted for meat identification. Mitochondrial 12s rRNA gene was also exploited so many workers with higher precision of result. Different PCR based methods can be used.

5.1 Restriction fragment length polymorphism (RFLP)

Polymerase chain reaction-restricted fragment length polymorphism (PCR-RFLP) is a modified form of PCR in which conserved target gene is amplified and resultant PCR product is digested with specific restriction endonuclease enzyme to get a restriction pattern or fingerprints (Partis *et al.,* 2000). This is also suitable method for identification of even degraded DNA with apomorphic sites. The first step in this technique is extraction of DNA polymerase and specific primers. It is suitable method for the analysis of very low amount of meat (1mg). It is a faster and more sensitive method than DNA hybridization. By this technique proper identification of male and females can be done by using PCR and genomic DNA extraction from raw muscles. It is not hundred per cent accurate methods because of existence of some intraspecific variability within the species as in the sheep, turkey and chicken meat.

5.1.1 Raw materials, chemicals, reagents and equipments require

- Sample extract, purified DNA, Taq DNA polymerase, PCR reaction mixture, dNTP mixture, forward and reverse primers, agarose gel, autoclaved water and assay buffer.
- Chloroform, phenolic Tris buffer (0.1 M Tris-base, pH 8.0), Isoamylalcohol, Ribonuclease-A, DNA lysis buffer (pH 8.0), Proteinase-K solution (20 mg/ml), 10 M ammonium acetate, ethanol, 1X Tris-EDTA buffer.
- Gradient PCR machine/thermal cycler, agarose gel electrophoresis unit, UV illumination, Gel Doc (Gel documentation system) and microfuge, dry bath, knife scissors, hot water bath, magnetic stirrer.

5.1.2 Preparation of DNA extract

- *For preparation sample extract follow the phenol:* chloroform method as described Sambrook and Russel (2001). The detail procedure is given as under:
- Collect muscle tissue sample carefully and remove all separable connective tissues, fat, fascia etc.
- Weigh 0.5 g tissue samples, cut into fine pieces and then homogenize with 10 volumes (w/v) of DNA lysis buffer (pH 8.0) containing Ribonuclease-A (20 μg/ml).
- Incubate the tubes at 37°C for 1 h.
- Add proteinase-K solution at 20 mg/ml concentration and incubate again at 50°C for 3 -4 h.
- Gently swirl the tubes intermittently and after incubation period is over add equal volumes of phenolic Tris buffer (0.1 M Tris-base, pH 8.0)
- Vortex the tubes for about 10 min and then centrifuge them at 1000 ×g for 15 min.

- Decant the aqueous layer into a separate tubes and add equal volume of phenol: chloroform: isoamylalcohol (25:24:1) solution, mix well and centrifuge again.
- *Collect the upper layer and add equal volume of phenol:* chloroform: isoamylalcohol (25:24:1) solution again and centrifuge.
- Collect upper layer into a separate tube and add equal volume of chloroform and then centrifuge.
- Collect upper layer again in to a fresh tube containing 0.2 volumes of 10 M ammonium acetate and 2 volumes of absolute ethanol.
- Mix well the content to precipitate the DNA.
- Centrifuge the tubes at 12500 ×g for 10 min; wash the DNA pellet twice with 70% alcohol by centrifugation at 12500 ×g for 5 min each.
- Let dry it in a dry bath at 60°C, dissolved in 50 µL 1X Tris-EDTA buffer.
- Store at -20°C until further use.

5.1.3 Procedure

- Perform PCR using 50 µL reaction mixture consisting of 5 µL of 10X assay buffer [160 mM $(NH4)_2SO_4$, 670 mM Tris-base, pH 8.8, 0.1% tween-20, 25 mM $MgCl_2$]; 1 µL 200µM of dNTP mix, 1µl of 20 pmol each of forward (5′-CCATCCAACATCTCAGC ATGATGAAA-3′ 26 mer) and reverse (5′-GCCCCTCAGAA TGATATTTGTCCTCA-3′ 20 mer) primers (Carr and Marshall, 1991), 2.0 U Taq DNA polymerase.
- Add 50 ng of purified DNA and autoclave water to make up the final volume.
- Spin the tubes for a brief.
- Keep the tubes in the PCR block and set the PCR condition as an initial denaturation for 94°C for 5 min followed by 35 cycles of denaturation at 94°C for 45s, primer annealing temperature at 60°C for 45s and 1 min elongation at 72°C (DNA synthesis) and a final extension for 10 min at 72°C.

- Hold the PCR products at 4°C.
- Purify of PCR amplified products using commercially available purification kit as per the protocol of the kit.
- Digest the PCR products with suitable restriction enzymes (*Alu* I, *Hinf* I, *Taq* I and *Rsa* I).
- Prepare enzyme buffer mix should contain 2 μL of 10X buffer and 1 μL of restriction enzyme (*Alu* I, *Hinf* I, *Rsa* I).
- Now prepare reaction mix using 10 μl of purified PCR product and 3 μl of enzyme buffer mix and make the volume upto 30 μl using autoclaved Milli Q water.
- Incubate the reaction mix at 37 °C for *Alu* I, *Hinf* I and *Rsa* I and 65 °C for *Taq* I for 12 h.
- Add 3 μl of loading dye to the above reaction mixture stop the enzyme activity.
- Prepare the agarose gel containing 2.5 % agarose in 1x TBE solution and before pouring in the gel casting frame add 0.5 μg/mL ethidium bromide.
- Place the comb for making wells and subsequently for loading the digested samples and 100pb ladder.
- Run the electrophoresis unit at 70 V for 2 h and visualize the amplified products under UV illumination and take a snap using gel documentation system.

Interpretation

Interpret the result based on the digested fragments (in bp) for PCR-RFLP

5.2 Species-specific PCR

- In this technique species-specific DNA in femto grams (fg) and pico grams (pg) can be detected in both processed and unprocessed meat samples by using targeted amplification of rRNA genes (12, 16, 18 S), actin-multigene which is highly conserved in eukaryotes, satellite DNA, cytochrome -b gene, cytochrome oxidase – II, growth hormone gene, melanocortnin gene, mt D-loop, myofibrillar components and satellite I DNA using PCR. By this technique very old samples even of more than 100 million years can also be identified.

5.2.1 Principle

- In this process in-vitro amplification of target DNA, a polymerase enzyme sythenises new DNA which is specific to the target using specific primers and other ingredients required for DNA synthesis. PCR produces millions of copies of target DNA in a span of 2-3 hours thereby producing DNA that could be documented thereby allowing meat speciation.

5.2.2 Raw materials, chemicals, reagents and equipments require

- Purified DNA (prepare following method as mentioned for RFLP), Taq DNA polymerase, PCR reaction mixture, dNTP mixture, forward and reverse primers, agarose gel, 100bp DNA ladder, 6X gel loading dye, autoclaved water and assay buffer.
- Chloroform, phenolic Tris buffer (0.1 M Tris-base, pH 8.0), Isoamylalcohol, Ribonuclease-A, DNA lysis buffer (pH 8.0), Proteinase-K solution (20 mg/ml), 10 M ammonium acetate, ethanol, 1X Tris-EDTA buffer.
- Gradient PCR machine/thermal cycler, agarose gel electrophoresis unit, UV illumination, Gel Doc (Gel documentation system) and microfuge, hot water bath, magnetic stirrer.

5.2.3 Procedure

- Perform PCR using 25 µL reaction mixture consisting of 2.5 µL of 10X assay buffer [160 mM $(NH4)_2SO_4$, 670 mM Tris-base, pH 8.8, 0.1% tween-20, 25 mM $MgCl_2$]; 0.25 µL 200µM of dNTP mix, 0.5 µl of 20 pmol each of forward and reverse primers; 1 U Taq DNA polymerase.
- Add 50 ng of purified DNA and autoclave water to make up the final volume.
- Spin the tubes for a brief.
- Keep the tubes in the PCR block and set the PCR condition as an initial denaturation for 95°C for 5 min followed by 30 cycles of denaturation at 95°C for 30s, primer annealing temperature at

55°C for 30s and 30s elongation at 72 °C (DNA synthesis) and a final extension for 5 min at 95°C.

- Hold the PCR products at 4°C.
- Prepare the agarose gel containing 2% agarose in 1x TBE solution and before pouring in the gel casting frame add 0.5 μg/mL ethidium bromide.
- Place the comb for making wells and subsequently for loading the amplified products (5μL) and 100 bp DNA ladder stained with 6X gel loading dye (1 μL).
- Run the electrophoresis unit at 40 – 60 V for 1 – 3 h and visualize the amplified products under UV illumination and take a snap using gel documentation system.

5.3 Multiplex PCR

5.3.1 Principle

- In this technique many targets are simultaneously amplified which helps in detection of many species in a short period of time (Matsunaga *et al.,* 1999). By this technique organ meat can also be detected like mixing of duck liver in goose liver can easily identified. For that purpose multiplex PCR with common forward and species –specific reverse primers to nuclear repeated target (5S rDNA gene) is used.

5.3.2 Raw materials, chemicals, reagents and equipments require

- Purified DNA(prepare following method as mentioned for RFLP), Taq DNA polymerase, PCR reaction mixture, dNTP mixture, forward and reverse primers, agarose gel, 100bp DNA ladder, 6X gel loading dye, autoclaved water and assay buffer.
- Chloroform, phenolic Tris buffer (0.1 M Tris-base, pH 8.0), Isoamylalcohol, Ribonuclease-A, DNA lysis buffer (pH 8.0), Proteinase-K solution (20 mg/ml), 10 M ammonium acetate, ethanol, 1X Tris-EDTA buffer.
- Gradient PCR machine/thermal cycler, agarose gel electrophoresis unit, UV illumination, Gel Doc (Gel documentation system) and microfuge, hot water bath, magnetic stirrer.

5.3.3 Procedure

- Perform PCR using 50 µL reaction mixture consisting of 5 µL of 10X assay buffer [160 mM $(NH4)_2SO_4$, 670 mM Tris-base, pH 8.8, 0.1% tween-20, 25 mM $MgCl_2$]; 2.5µL 10 mM of dNTP mix, 1 µl of 20 pmol each of forward and reverse primers; 3 U Taq DNA polymerase.
- Add 50 ng of purified DNA and autoclave water to make up the final volume.
- Spin the tubes for a brief.
- Optimize the multiplex reaction mixture by using species-specific reverse primers at different ratios viz. goat: chicken: beef: sheep: pig: horse: :0.3:2.5:0.5:2.5:0.5:1.8.
- Keep the tubes in the PCR block and set the PCR condition as an initial denaturation for 94°C for 5 min followed by 33 cycles of denaturation at 94°C for 45s, primer annealing temperature at 61°C for 45s and 45s elongation at 72 °C (DNA synthesis) and a final extension for 10 min at 72°C.
- Hold the PCR products at 4°C.
- Prepare the agarose gel containing 3% agarose in 0.5x TBE buffer, heat the solution until get transparent, cool to 60 °C, add and 10 µl of ethidium bromide (1:10 diluted 20 mg/ml), mix thoroughly and then pour up to 4 mm thickness of the gel.
- Allow the gel to set and remove the comb gently.
- Submerge the casted gel along with the running tray in the electrophoresis tank containing 1.0X TBE buffer.
- Mix a volume of 6 µl of PCR product with 2 µl of 6X gel loading dye and then load into the well.
- Load a 100 bp DNA ladder in the separate well.
- Run the electrophoresis unit at 60–70 V for 2 h and visualize the amplified products under UV illumination and take a snap using gel documentation system.

Interpretation

- Interpret the result taking into consideration of ladder size (bp) corresponding to the size of the amplicons for goat, chicken, cattle, sheep, pig and horse of 157, 227, 274, 331, 398 and 439 bp, respectively.

5.4 Forensically informative nucleotide sequencing (FINS)

- In this technique conserved region of gene specific to a species is amplified and the PCR product is cloned, sequenced and the sequences are analysed (Kocher *et al.*, 1989). For this purpose 12S rRNA gene sequence analyses is the most preferred method for differentiation of beef, buffalo meat, mutton and chevon.

5.4.1 Principle

- Conserved region of DNA sequnces provide information in the algorithm of ATGC which determines origin of species.

5.4.2 Raw materials, chemicals, reagents and equipments require

- Purified DNA (prepare following method as mentioned for RFLP), Taq DNA polymerase, PCR reaction mixture, dNTP mixture, forward and reverse primers, agarose gel, autoclaved water and assay buffer.
- Chloroform, phenolic Tris buffer (0.1 M Tris-base, pH 8.0), Isoamylalcohol, Ribonuclease-A, DNA lysis buffer (pH 8.0), Proteinase-K solution (20 mg/ml), 10 M ammonium acetate, ethanol, 1X Tris-EDTA buffer.
- Gradient PCR machine/thermal cycler, agarose gel electrophoresis unit, UV illumination, Gel Doc (Gel documentation system) and microfuge, hot water bath, magnetic stirrer.

5.4.3 Procedure

- Perform PCR using 50 μL reaction mixture consisting of 5 μL of 10X assay buffer [160 mM $(NH_4)2SO_4$, 670 mM Tris-base, pH 8.8, 0.1% tween-20, 25 mM $MgCl_2$]; 1 μL 200μM of dNTP mix, 1μl of 20 pmol each of forward (5′-CAA ACT GGG ATT AGA TAC CCC ACT AT-3′ 26 mer) and reverse (5′- GAG GGT GAC GGG CGG TGT GT-3′ 20 mer) primers; 1.66 U Taq DNA polymerase.
- Add 50 μg of purified DNA and autoclave water to make up the final volume.
- Spin the tubes for a brief.

- Keep the tubes in the PCR block and set the PCR condition as an initial denaturation for 94°C for 5 min followed by 30 cycles of denaturation at 94°C for 45s, primer annealing temperature at 60°C for 45s and 1 min elongation at 72 °C (DNA synthesis) and a final extension for 5 min at 72°C.
- Hold the PCR products at 4°C.
- Prepare the agarose gel containing 2% agarose in 1x TBE solution and before pouring in the gel casting frame add 0.5 μg/mL ethidium bromide.
- Place the comb for making wells and subsequently for loading the amplified products.
- Run the electrophoresis unit at 50 V for 2 h and visualize the amplified products under UV illumination and take a snap using gel documentation system.
- **Sequencing of PCR products from mt 12S rRNA gene Sequence**

  The PCR products using automatic DNA sequencer at a DNA sequencing facility. Align the sequences using *'Megalign"* and compare by *'Clustal'* method (DNAstar, Inc. 1996), or any other equivalent software.
- **BLAST analysis of mt 12S rRNA gene sequence**
  - Log in to the NCBI site (http://www.ncbi.nlm.nih.gov/blast/Blast.cgi).
  - Select the nucleotide blast (*BlastN*).
  - Enter the unknown sequence (Accession number, gi, or FASTA).
  - Select and collect the highly similar nucleotide sequences (*Megablast*).
  - Blast the sequence.
  - Retrieve the data in two modes, i.e., distance tree and alignments.
- **Distance tree of results:** Search the sequence by its ID, taxonomic name, sequence title or the Blast name. If necessary, browse a focus sub-tree as well as the alignment report of the desired species (or accessions).

- In *'Alignments'* option, the sequence show significant alignments along with their accession numbers, title, score, E (bits) value, followed by the detailed information about the length of sequence, percent identity, gaps, etc.

Interpretation

- Interpret the result based on the distance tree and alignments with the query sequence, the nearest species with the maximum score was found and the animal species is identified.

References

Carr, S. M. and Marshall, H. D. 1991. *Can. Bull. Fish. Aquat. Sci./ Bull. Can. Sci. Halieut. Aquat.* 48 (1): 48-52.

Kocher *et al.* 1989. *Proc. Natl. Acad. Sci. U.S.A.* 86: 6196-6200.

Matsunaga, T. *et al.* 1999. *Meat Science.* 51: 143-148.

Nagappa *et al.* 2010. *Veterinarski Arhiv.* 80 (5): 653-661.

Nagappa *et al.* 2011. *European Food Research and Technology.* 233:985-989.

Nagappa *et al.* 2011. *Small Ruminant Research.* 100: 153-158.

Nagappa *et al.* 2011. *Journal of Food Quality*, 34 (2): 142–149.

Nagappa S. Karabasanavar. 2008. Ph.D Thesis Submitted to the Govind Ballabh Pant University of Agriculture and Technology, Pantnagar, Uttarakhand, India.

Partis *et al.* 2000. *Meat Science.* 54: 369-376.

Sambrook, J. and Russell, D. W. 2001. Molecular cloning: A Laboratory Manual. 3rd edition. Cold Spring Harbour Laboratory Press, Cold Spring Harbour, New York.

Website: http://www.ncbi.nlm.nih.gov/blast

❑❑❑